Food Combining for Health

Don't mix foods that fight

by
Doris Grant and Jean Joice

Thorsons
An Imprint of HarperCollinsPublishers

Thorsons
An Imprint of HarperCollins*Publishers*
77–85 Fulham Palace Road,
Hammersmith, London W6 8JB

First published October 1984
Thirtieth Impression 1990
First mass market edition 1991
17 19 18

© Doris Grant and Jean Joice 1984, 1989, 1991
© John Mills 1984

Doris Grant and Jean Joice assert the moral right to
be identified as the authors of this work

A catalogue record for this book
is available from the British Library

ISBN 0 7225 2506 0

Printed in Great Britain by
HarperCollinsManufacturing Glasgow

FOOD COMBINING
FOR HEALTH

A fresh look at an established and successful system
of combining compatible foods to help prevent and
cure many of the diseases of Western civilization.

CONTENTS

PART FOUR: RECIPES FOR STARCH MEALS

ACKNOWLEDGEMENTS

We should like to thank Dr Jeannie Stirrat for so tire-lessly extracting for us during the past seven years many pertinent and helpful items from her medical journals and papers.

We should also like to thank Mrs Gordon Clemetson OBE, Dr John Breakwell and Dr Hugh Cox for sparing time to read this book in manuscript and for their continuing interest and encouragement.

Our gratitude is owed to the editors of the Hay System News of the 1930s for much valuable material and to the editors of *Healthy Living* and *Here's Health* for publishing Doris Grant's articles on the Hay System; it was the enormous interest these created that prompted the writing of this book.

Finally we should like to thank Pamela Kelly for her immense patience in typing and retyping the many amendments to the recipes, and Anthea Gordon for producing an impeccably consistent typescript from two very different styles.

FOREWORD

by Sir John Mills CBE

I am delighted to know that the Hay Diet is being resuscitated after all these years. I have a copy of the original book, which my sister, Annette, gave me over forty years ago, and on the flyleaf is written 'John Mills' Bible. Please do not remove'.

In 1942 I was invalided out of the Army with a man-size duodenal ulcer. In hospital I was fed on the usual ulcer-sufferer's diet of rice puddings, mashed potatoes etc., and after three months there was no improvement. In fact everything seized up and I became a walking zombie.

My sister, Annette, suggested to my wife, Mary, that she should put me immediately onto the Hay Diet and my first meal, which I remember with gratitude, was a thin minute steak, a large mixed salad and a small glass of claret. From that moment I have never looked back. After six weeks I was able to start work on a film.

Most diets, I find, are crashing bores, especially to hostesses, but if one follows the Hay Diet it is possible to go to any dinner, public or private, and offend no-one. All one has to remember is the principle of not mixing starch with protein. So one can wade one's way happily through any festive occasion until it comes to the sweet course. I find the best way of coping with this is to leave the sweet untouched, and the waiter will finally remove it, and nobody will have noticed.

I am sure that I could not, at my advanced age, cope with the work I have on hand at the moment if I were not a 'believer'. I am playing eight shows a week in *Little Lies* at Wyndham's Theatre, and the last Act is a marathon. It is essential that I am really fit, and for this I rely practically entirely on the Hay Diet. I am, incidentally, today wearing the jacket which I had made in 1938. It has not been let out, and I can still do the button up without any problem.

I wish the book every success, and I guarantee that anyone who follows the advice in it will derive the greatest of benefits from it.

INTRODUCTION

A Personal Experience

As we eat even so are we; our health is made or marred with our feet under the dinner table

Food Combining for Health was first published in October 1984. Three months later it became a runaway bestseller as grateful and enthusiastic readers spread the word amongst their relatives and friends. Evidence of the success of the Hay lifestyle is constantly confirmed by the letters we receive, and today, over six years after the book's publication, it continues to appear in bestseller lists and in feature articles in newspapers and magazines.

By January 1986 it was arousing such interest that the Cumberland Hotel in London opened a buffet serving delicious Hay System lunches. The book has also created great interest abroad and, apart from an American edition selling in the USA and Canada, it has been published in Dutch, Spanish, Portuguese, Hebrew, Greek, Serbo-Croat and Finnish.

This is a wonderful tribute to the efficacy of the Hay System, and its success is constantly confirmed by countless letters that Jean and I receive from converts. Many claim that it has changed their lives — in some cases miraculously. Knowing that the Hay System does not 'cure' but merely allows the body to heal itself, we are continually amazed at the extraordinary inbuilt healing powers of the body revealed in these letters, and the unbelievable speed with which they often work. Readers report agonizing arthritic pains removed within two weeks; allergies and psoriasis of long standing completely gone in four days; chronic migraine and hay fever banished in a matter of weeks; two pounds of excess weight shed in one week without counting calories or feeling hungry. Many more similar cases have been reported.

It was the efficacy and speed with which the Hay System resolved my own health problems that turned me into a lifelong follower. In my late twenties severely painful rheumatoid trouble in my joints nearly crippled me and took all the fun out of life. When all the usual medical therapies had been applied with no effect whatsoever, a doctor-cousin came to the rescue with a very unorthodox prescription. It consisted of three columns of foods — proteins, starches and acid fruits — accompanied with the instruction: 'Don't mix foods that fight!'

By the end of just one week this unusual prescription, conscientiously carried out, produced a totally unexpected bonus: the complete termination of nagging indigestion pains which had plagued me for fifteen years. After another week there were more unexpected results: an ability to think more clearly than formerly and a great general feeling of well-being which inspired me to carry on. By the end of four weeks all the rheumatoid pains had gone and have never returned (I am now 86).

After a year I felt like a new woman. I was tireless and filled with a new energy that I had never before experienced. The more difficult the task the more I welcomed it as a challenge to my newly-found health and abilities. Yet, apart from not eating meat or acid fruits (apples, oranges, pears, grapefruit, etc.) with bread or sugared foods at the same meal, there had been no other change in my diet. I knew nothing whatsoever about wholefoods, and was still eating white bread and refined sugar, to whose potential dangers I had not been alerted. This fact is of the highest significance; it provided unique evidence that 'not mixing foods that fight' really works. It also demolishes the claim by sceptics that any benefit derived from the Hay System is entirely due to a changeover to wholefood eating. During the past forty years I have received many letters from life-long wholefooders who had been unable to resolve their health problems until adopting the Hay lifestyle.

Towards the end of my first year of compatible eating I discovered and carefully read Dr William Howard Hay's inspiring book *A New Health Era*, and I found that there was much more to the Hay System than 'not mixing foods that fight'. As a result of reading this book my diet improved still further. I felt I had set out on a marvellous adventure. I have to admit, though, that departing from orthodox eating habits was not at first a rose-strewn path. Relations and friends, especially medical friends, pooh-poohed the idea of any connection between food and health, and thought I had taken leave of my senses, whereas I was, in fact, just beginning to come to them. Friends argued that I was going to miss out on all the joys of eating: 'What, no sugar? — no biscuits and cheese? — no apple tart? You poor thing!'

I found, however, that this way of eating was in no sense a wearisome, calorie-counting diet of constant self-denial, but was instead a delicious way of eating which ensures health and fitness, and minimizes the necessity for medical treatment. The fitter I became, the more convinced I was that *we hold our health in our own hands to a very large extent*.

By the end of four years of compatible eating I produced a much longed-for second child *nine years after my first-born*, despite warnings from doctor and gynaecologist after this first birth that *I could never have any more children*; there had been serious complications after an emergency Caesarian operation. But they had reckoned without the healing powers of compatible eating! Moreover, the second birth, according to the gynaecologist, was a 'textbook demonstration of a beautifully normal birth'!

By the end of another three years I had proof in plenty of these healing powers, while writing long weekly articles on the Hay System for a well-known national Sunday newspaper — the now defunct *Sunday Graphic* — in 1936 and 1937. These articles continued for nine months and generated enormous interest, bringing into the *Graphic* office hundreds of letters every week.

The letters were an education, and most revealing: their almost monotonous burden was the virtually complete failure of medical treatment as far as the degenerative diseases were concerned; the 'wonder drugs' never effected the hoped-for cure. Often there were recitals of complete disaster in treatment, and of the 'cure' being far worse than the disease, frequently proving fatal.

As the weeks and months passed, however, there were many accounts from followers of the articles, of greatly improved health. The benefits of the Hay System were often felt even within the first week. There were also reports of increased zest for living; depression replaced by optimism; digestion pains eliminated; freedom from colds; arthritic pains lessened and movement freer; and constipation a thing of the past. Many readers reported great relief from tiredness and chronic sleeplessness. One of the most unforgettable letters was from a woman of seventy who wrote: 'I feel well for the first time in my life!'

These accounts provided convincing proof of Dr Hay's contention: that the primary cause of disease is not the outside germ which always gets the blame, but the inside state of the body-soil, created mainly by wrong living habits and wrong eating habits.

The explanation for all this lies in the fact that the Hay System removes the obstacles, created by these habits, which prevent the inbuilt healing powers of the body from restoring perfect health and wholeness. In other words, the Hay System allows the body to heal itself.

The tremendous interest that this book has aroused, and the superior health and fitness that so many followers are now enjoying — some for the first time in their lives — is a reflection of the worldwide interest in healthy eating today. It would appear that Dr Hay's 'new health era' is now well and truly with us.

DORIS GRANT

PART ONE
THE THEORY AND THE PROOF
by
Doris Grant

1.

A GREAT PIONEER

William Howard Hay was born in Hartstown, Pennsylvania, U.S.A., in 1866. Prophet, philosopher, hard-pan Presbyterian of Scottish stock, he grew up from early boyhood with the sole thought of medicine as a calling.

He was especially fortunate that both his parents were of exceptional character; his father, according to Dr Hay, 'was possessed of an unusually fine mind, was a great reader of good literature and developed into one of the solid men of his community.' His mother 'combined with a very excellent education the Scottish characteristics of thrift and industry, with also one of the most even dispositions imaginable, an ability to see through a great many things that looked difficult to others and a sense of right and wrong that knew absolutely no compromise.' Dr Hay was richly endowed with his parents' fine characteristics, and these undoubtedly provided him with the courage and strength of character to overcome the heartbreaking difficulties which beset him when his unorthodox treatment of disease evoked the enmity of his profession.

He graduated from the University of New York on 26 March 1891. For the next sixteen years he practised medicine 'according to the best light of his time', and did much surgery. At the end of this period he broke down in health, proving, as he admitted, 'that he knew as little as the rest of the predisposing causes of disease.' He became very ill, developed Bright's disease, with high blood pressure, and finally a dilated heart. For this latter condition there was no relief in medicine, or at least only temporary relief. He thought his career was over, and received a warning from his doctors to put his affairs in order.

Inspiration

In *A New Health Era* Dr Hay related how this warning inspired him to treat his own symptoms. He did so by 'eating fundamentally', as he called it, eating 'only such things as he believed were intended by nature as food for man, taking them in natural form, and in quantities no greater than seemed necessary for his present need.' (It is interesting to note that sixty years later, Surgeon Capt. T.L. Cleave was to put forward similar concepts in his book *The Saccharine Disease*.) To the great astonishment of Dr Hay's doctors his symptoms gradually disappeared, and at the end of three months he felt fitter and stronger than he had done for many years. He reduced his weight — he had been greatly overweight — from 225 lbs to 175 lbs and soon was able to run long distances without distress.

This experience, he wrote, deepened the conviction that had been growing over the past sixteen years *that medicine was on the wrong track*; it was merely fussing with the end results of a condition instead of attempting to remove the cause, 'for here was his own case recovering from a condition that the best authorities said was incurable.' It had taken a major health disaster and a hopeless outlook for the future to open his eyes to the possibility of treating disease along dietary lines, unorthodox although these at first seemed.

It was not, however, till the middle of 1908 that he had regenerated himself to his own satisfaction. By 1911 Dr Hay was virtually certain that he had discovered a 'surefire treatment' for diabetes. He little realized then that this same treatment would prove equally efficacious in the treatment of all disease.

For the next four years he devoted all his time to

treating his patients along dietary lines in order to prove or disprove his contention that we are exactly what we eat and 'that the body is merely a composite of what goes into it daily in the form of food and drink.' These four years provided proof in plenty that his contention was right and that anyone can be as well as desired if given the right food in the right way (provided, of course, there has been no serious, irreversible organic change). Thus he developed over the years the system of eating for which he became famous. He always claimed, however, that *he had not discovered anything new*, but had merely used the knowledge already made public by others and consolidated it, adding his own deep convictions with a dash of common sense. Moreover, he made no claims that he 'cured' any disease, and emphasized that this system merely removed the obstacles in the way of nature's own marvellous healing powers.

The message in *A New Health Era* was simple: that no matter how diverse are our diseases, there is one underlying cause — wrong chemical conditions in the body. These conditions are created through the manufacture and accumulation of acid end-products of digestion and metabolism in amounts greater than the body can eliminate. A state then develops 'that is variously called auto-intoxication, acid-autotoxicosis,' toxaemia, self-poisoning, or whatever you like to call it.' This results in a lowering of the body's vital alkaline reserve leading, in turn, to departure from health. 'The science of medicine takes no cognizance of this accumulation,' wrote Dr Hay, 'till disease, that is definite pathology, has developed.'

He taught his patients that there were four main causes of the accumulation of acid end-products of digestion: eating too much meat; over-consumption of refined carbohydrates — white flour products, refined sugar, and refined carbohydrates of any kind; disregard for the laws of chemistry as these apply to the digestion of foods; and constipation.

Dr Hay also taught his patients that although many people, especially young people, build up a tolerance to incompatible mixtures just as people build up a tolerance for increasing doses of irritant poisons, they do so at a very considerable and continuing cost in vitality. This formed tolerance, he warned, is unnatural. But if compatible eating is followed long enough, it can be removed. Then, claimed Dr Hay, 'you cannot go back to the practice of mixing starches and proteins without immediate notice from your stomach that you have made a mistake — one that you are not likely to repeat.' He promised that two weeks would be sufficient to convince anyone of this, and that the reward for the effort would be greatly improved vitality and health.

Dr Hay never forgot to teach the importance of other adjuvants to health — fresh air, exercise, daily baths, sunshine, and rest. Nor did he forget to teach the importance of health to the spiritual man: 'When the body and mind are in harmony, only then will there be an opportunity for proper spiritual development; for do not forget that the spiritual man is the first man, the mental man the second, and the physical the third man; and only when these second and third are in harmony can there be a proper spiritual state.'

Disbelief

In spite of the ease and speed with which anyone could prove for himself the truth of the starch-protein concept, the Hay System received a battering of criticism.

The bitterest attacks came from Dr Hay's fellow physicians. The teaching of the means of preventing disease had not, in Dr Hay's time, caught on with the medical profession, simply because their entire teaching had been (and still is) directed towards the *treatment* of disease, not its *prevention*. Dr Hay's teaching was therefore stark heresy and naturally condemned as such.

As he became more and more convinced of the truth of his findings, so his colleagues became more and more sceptical. Ironically, while realizing success in his treatment of disease beyond his wildest hopes, restoring to normal health countless cases termed hopeless by the highest of medical authorities, he found himself written off as a simple quack. His frustration must have been immense when, armed not only with an inspired idea but also with proof of its truth, he was met with a blank wall of disbelief and incomprehension.

The medical profession was most certainly not ready for Dr Hay's concepts. At that time doctors were fervent apostles of 'the germ theory of disease.' They were also enthusiasts for the new wonder-drug era which promised 'a pill for every ill'; so they believed that there was no need whatsoever for nutritional therapy. His concepts were rejected with scorn and he was constantly subjected to the vehement opposition of entrenched orthodoxy, even to slander, libel, and the most diabolical of rumours. But he was a courageous man who never faltered in defending his beliefs and in countering all opposition with lucid and reasoned arguments, never losing his temper or his strong sense of humour. The latter attribute, and his great personal charm, endeared him to his patients and to all who had the good fortune to hear him lecture.

It is significant that many physicians attended his lectures in both England and Scotland, and many of these spoke to Dr Hay afterwards and said they were in full accord with everything he taught. Some admitted that they were students of the Hay System and were using it in their work with their patients. Many, moreover, told of results which could not have been achieved in any other way, except by applying the system with real understanding.

Dr Hay died in 1940, at the age of seventy-four, a year after a serious accident, sadly, just as medical thinking was beginning to appreciate the important relationship of nutrition to health.

Vindication

That Dr Hay was 'a prophet way ahead of his time' has now been fully confirmed by the vast change in attitude towards nutrition today by many of the foremost medical authorities in both the U.S.A. and Great Britain. Despite all the marvels of modern medicine, despite the wonder drugs and the astronomical cost of our health services, the health of both nations is deteriorating and disease is attacking at an ever-increasingly early age. Medical authorities are now frankly admitting that medicine is on the wrong track and are urging a switch of emphasis from curative medicine to preventive medicine — to dealing with the *causes* of disease instead of merely treating *the symptoms*. As a result, nutrition is now being promoted as the chief priority in preventive medicine. In fact attention is now being focused as never before on the close relationship of nutrition to health, *and on just such concepts as were held sixty years ago by Dr William Howard Hay, gifted surgeon and general practitioner of note*. Witness the following signs and portents:

● Since the 1950s, the research and writings on human ecology of a number of medical scientists have produced evidence of the close connection between refined carbohydrates and chemically adulterated foods and such diverse symptoms as allergies, depression, migraine, fatigue, skin diseases, schizophrenia, and uncontrolled aggressive behaviour in children. The research, in particular, of Dr Théron Randolph and Dr Ben Feingold in the U.S.A., and of Dr Richard Mackarness in Great Britain, has been outstanding. They are nevertheless having the same bitter battle for recognition by orthodox medicine as had Dr Hay fifty years ago.

● A society formed in 1967, The McCarrison Society, whose members consist of doctors, surgeons, dentists, veterinary surgeons, and community health workers, is pledged 'to advance education in, and initiate, carry out and sponsor, research into the relationship between nutrition and health . . .' The Society was named after the internationally-acclaimed British nutritional pioneer, the late Sir Robert McCarrison, whose book *Nutrition and Health* (McCarrison Society, 1982) should be mandatory reading for all health-conscious people. Dr Hay claimed that he owed much to McCarrison's teachings.

● In 1968, the validity of the germ theory of disease was seriously questioned for the first time in a leading British medical journal. In *The Lancet* of 18 May, Professor G.T. Stewart revealed its weaknesses in a revolutionary paper: 'Dogma Disputed, Limitations of the Germ Theory'. Prof. Stewart's message was, in effect, that acceptance of the germ theory as the main cause of infectious disease has been responsible for orthodox medicine overlooking other more important, or equally important, causes such as genetic and metabolic effects, behaviour (smoking etc.), and *certain nutritional deficiencies*.

● In the 1970s, an epoch-making book, *The Saccharine Disease* by Surgeon Capt. T.L. Cleave, started off the present revolutionary medical preoccupation with bran and 'fibre', nutrition and preventive medicine. It postulated one common cause of many of the present-day degenerative diseases — the consumption of *refined carbohydrates*. Moreover, it has become the major reference work for the growing number of medical specialists throughout the world who believe — as Dr Hay did — that our twentieth-century diet is responsible for the vast amount of disease in today's society.

● Also in the 1970s, another important book, *The Role of Medicine: Dream, Mirage or Nemesis*, by Professor Thomas McKeown, contained the blunt message that more attention should now be paid to nutrition, and that the modifications of the conditions which lead to disease will achieve more than any medical intervention after the illness has begun. That, too, was Dr Hay's message.

● In 1972 the Editor of the *British Medical Journal* exhorted: 'We now have to learn the more subtle relationships that exist between nutrition and medicine, and how change in food habits and change in methods of food preparation may affect health. *Medical education must keep pace with the rapid advance in this subject.*'

● In 1977, this same editor wrote: 'Enthusiasm for fibre is sweeping the world. The journals are full of it, the popular press revels in it, and doctors take time off from prescribing it only to attend international conferences on it . . . in "discovering" fibre modern man is waking up to the fact that his food is systematically deprived of fibre on its journey from field to grocery shop.'

● Also in 1977, the Editor of *The Lancet* stated: 'About five years ago dietary fibre burst into the consciousness of the medical world, having smouldered at the back of some minds for decades.'

● In 1981, the consumer magazine *Which?* discovered in its researches that more people than ever are clamouring for drugless treatment. (This, however, is not sufficient — people must also be willing *to assume responsibility for keeping themselves fit*.)

● In 1982, on 14 December, at the British Medical

Association's 150th Annual Dinner, H.R.H. Prince Charles affirmed, in his presidential speech, with reference to drugs: 'Wonderful as many of them are, it should be more widely stressed by doctors that the health of human beings is so often determined by their behaviour, their food, and the nature of their environment.'

● In January 1983, in *Homoeopathy Today*, a doctor wrote that he advised his patients 'not to eat high proteins with high carbohydrate foods', and stressed the importance to health of recognizing the trinity of mind, body, and spirit.

● Also in 1983, remarkably, the potential for health of 'fringe medicine', now elevated to the status of 'Alternative Medicine', was being considered by a new research committee. *Hospital Doctor* of 14 April reported that 'Alternative Medicine' is to be 'put under the scientific spotlight' by the Research Council for Complementary Medicine, consisting of both conventional and alternative specialists. This Council has been formed 'because of growing public interest in acupuncture, homoeopathy and herbalism.' The committee believe that it will 'help to stop the erosion of public confidence in orthodox medicine.'

● Finally, in June 1983, in his speech on stepping down as president of the British Medical Association, H.R.H. Prince Charles urged: 'Don't over-estimate the sophisticated approach to medicine. It seems that account has to be taken of those sometimes long-neglected complementary methods of medicine.'

It would seem his message has had the desired effect. On Wednesday 17 August 1983, the national press announced that in a revolutionary move, the B.M.A. was launching an enquiry into all forms of alternative medicine and that some may soon become available on the Health Service. In the *Daily Mail* John Illman wrote: 'The move marks a remarkable about-turn for the B.M.A., which for years has resisted what has been regarded as "quack medicine" . . . the background to the B.M.A. move is the growing interest in Britain in health matters and preventive measures against illness.'

In this same article John Illman quoted Dr Malcolm Carruthers, author of *The Western Way of Death*: 'There is a crisis of confidence in drugs. No medical system can afford not to take account of the public's desire to play a larger part in determining their own medical treatment.'

John Illman also quoted Dr Anthony Fry, consultant physician in psychological medicine at Guy's Hospital: 'As a profession we have spent too much time giving Valium instead of teaching patients how to relax. *We spend too much time treating symptoms and not causes.*' (My emphasis — D.G.) *So affirmed Dr William Howard Hay, sixty years ahead of his time, throughout all his writings.*

What better vindication could this prophet have than the decision of the British Medical Association to launch an enquiry into alternative medicine?

A New Health Era

It would appear from these 'signs and portents' that the 'new health era' so dear to Dr Hay's heart has indeed begun. If this book contributes to this era, even in a small way, by helping its readers to achieve greater health and happiness, its authors will perhaps have repaid a small part of the great debt they both owe Dr Hay for countless benefits received from his teachings. How better to end this chapter than in his own words:

To really live is to be in exuberant health continually, and when in that condition nothing palls on one, nothing is devoid of interest, and life is the swellest job in the world. When in splendid health every breath we draw is filled with inspiration, everything we do is full of interest, there are so many things to do, so much to accomplish, so many delectable prospects in life that even if we are poor and unknown we still may fully enjoy life, for life is a splendid thing if we are really alive.

2.

THE HAY SYSTEM EXPLAINED

There is nothing so powerful as an idea whose time has come.

The Hay System consists of five important rules:

1. Starches and sugars should not be eaten with proteins and acid fruits at the same meal.
2. Vegetables, salads and fruits should form the major part of the diet.
3. Proteins, starches and fats should be eaten in small quantities.
4. Only whole grain and unprocessed starches should be used, and all refined processed foods should be taboo — in particular, white flour and sugar and all foods made with them, and highly processed fats such as margarine.
5. An interval of at least four to four-and-a-half hours should elapse between meals of different character.

The cardinal rule of the Hay System, not mixing carbohydrates (i.e., starches and sugars) with proteins and acid fruits, is generally misunderstood, although based on sound physiological principles long existing and long forgotten. In order to understand this rule it is therefore necessary to explain the classification of carbohydrates and proteins in the context of compatible food combinations:

The proteins are concentrated (20 per cent or more) animal proteins such as meat, fish, cheese, poultry.

The carbohydrates are concentrated (20 per cent or more)

starches, such as grains, bread and cereals, potatoes; and sugars.

Misunderstanding regarding this classification has been the main reason why many investigators have dismissed the starch-protein concept as being without foundation. The main argument put forward to refute this concept is that nature herself combines proteins and starches in most foods; that if it is wrong to combine these dissimilar elements at the same meal then nature herself is in error.

On first glance this argument would seem to be unanswerable; it is widely acknowledged that nature does not make mistakes.

On second glance this argument reveals shallow thinking; nature does not combine in one food *a high concentration* of protein (as in meat) with *a high concentration* of starch (as in grains). Although meats do contain carbohydrate, this is in the form of glycogen which requires little, if any, digestion, and its presence therefore does not interfere with the conditions necessary for protein digestion. Similarly, although grains contain about 10 per cent protein, this is incomplete in character, and is not in a concentrated form (as in meat); its presence therefore does not interfere with the conditions necessary for starch digestion.

Apart from the single exception of the mature, or dried, legumes — peas, beans, lentils and peanuts — nature combines starches and proteins in the same food in a form and in proportions which digest together perfectly, and in such a way, also, that the food is either predominantly starch or predominantly protein. The dried legumes are 'the exception which proves the rule'; they contain too high a percentage of both protein and starch to be compatible in themselves (but become compatible and highly beneficial when sprouted — see Part Two). People who are accustomed to their habitual consumption over a long period can build up a tolerance to them just as they can build up a tolerance, for example, to smoking. But anyone who is not accustomed to them usually experiences discomfort — and very audible protests from his digestive organs!

The Why and How of Starch and Protein Digestion
Proteins require an acid medium for digestion. When animal proteins enter into the stomach this stimulates the production of hydrochloric acid which activates the enzyme pepsin, whose function is the splitting and digesting of the proteins. This action in the stomach can only take place in a wholly acid medium; the presence of any high starch or sugar with its accompanying alkalis interferes with, or neutralizes, this acid medium, and the proteins are then incompletely digested. The implications of this incomplete protein digestion are more serious than has hitherto been suspected. This is discussed in Chapter Three, in relation to allergy.

Carbohydrates (starches and sugars) require an alkaline medium for digestion. This is initiated in the mouth by the action of the enzyme, ptyalin, which splits the starches into lower forms before entrance into the small intestine where their further reduction *and main digestion* takes place. As the whole process of starch digestion depends on its proper initiation in the mouth, all starch foods must be thoroughly chewed, otherwise the small intestine, although alkaline in all its secretions, cannot complete what the ptyalin started higher up in the tract.

The stomach acts as a mixing chamber in which the saliva, with its active ptyalin, is thoroughly incorporated into the starches. During this early sojourn in the stomach, lasting about thirty to forty-five minutes, the normal acidity of the stomach is insufficient to cancel out, or interfere with, the alkaline medium necessary for preparing the starches for their intestinal digestion. The presence of meat, however, or other acid-compelling foods, or acid fruits, arrests this preparation and fermentation follows; the splitting-down process of starches can only occur in a positive alkalinity.

When asked what was the scientific basis for the theory that starches and sugars should not be eaten with proteins and acid fruits at the same meal, Dr Hay replied:

> If starches are taken combined with acid fruits and if the stomach contents are withdrawn at intervals during digestion, it will be observed that the action of ptyalin has ceased and that the starches are not being split but will give the intense blue reaction of iodide of starch when iodine is applied to the chyme removed from the stomach. The same test may be performed with a combination of starches and proteins — the extraction of parts of chyme at intervals, as they happen during our digestion, will always show this arrest of ptyalin digestion meaning that the starches then unsplit will never be properly split.

For many years the teaching has been that the highest levels of acidity are in the resting stomach. This belief has been responsible for the advice given year after year, and still given to ulcer sufferers 'to avoid letting the stomach get empty.' But a number of authorities disagree with this belief (now in disrepute in certain medical quarters), including the physiologist A.H. James. In *Physiology of Gastric Digestion* (Arnold, London, 1957) he states: 'The highest acidities of all are reached *during the digestion of food, not when the stomach is empty.'*

This fact supports Dr Hay's contention that if no protein accompanies a starch food entering a resting stomach the amount of hydrochloric acid is insufficient *at first* to fully neutralize or overcome the alkalinity of the saliva present.

In 1936, the work of three Philadelphia investigators provided interesting laboratory confirmation of the starch-protein concept. In *Man Alive, You're Half Dead*!

(Bartholomew House Inc., 1956), Dr Daniel Munro gives an account of a study on five subjects by these investigators showing the degree of acidity in the stomach after protein meals, after starch meals, and after combined protein and starch meals. This study revealed that, one and a quarter hours after these meals were eaten, the stomach contents were most acid after the high protein meal, least acid after the high starch meal, and half way between both states after the mixed meal. Moreover, when the mixed meal was eaten it was clear that the proteins were being digested under difficulties as the acidity present was far lower than that shown as required by the all-protein meal and had actually been cut to one-third less by the presence of the starches and their accompanying alkalis.

This investigation clearly shows that when high starches and high proteins are mixed at one meal there is too much acid to permit the continued alkaline reduction of the starch part, and not enough acid to start the digestion of the protein part.

The usual teaching, however, is that when we eat food *of any kind* (such as proteins and starches) we produce gastric juice which contains hydrochloric acid. The answer, here, is that hydrochloric acid is stimulated in exact ratio to the amount of protein presented by the digestive task. This was shown by Pavlov's classic observations on dogs in *The Work of the Digestive Glands* (Charles Griffin & Co. Ltd, 1910).

As already pointed out, the protein in starches such as grains is both very small (about 10 per cent) and incomplete in character, and therefore does not stimulate sufficient hydrochloric acid to interfere, *for the first thirty to forty-five minutes*, with the alkaline medium necessary for the digestion of starches. During this time, the saliva — which has a pH value of 6.6, as compared with the pH 0.9 of pure gastric juice — acts as a natural buffer of the gastric acid.

Some physiologists and physicians disagree with Dr

Hay's explanation of the starch-protein theory and claim that the gastric acid is *necessary* for the splitting of the starches; the starch is often contained in protein 'envelopes' which require the acid for digestion so that the starch can be released. This claim is undoubtedly correct but it does not alter the fact that starches have a preliminary digestion in an *alkaline* medium which buffers the gastric acid for the first thirty to forty minutes in the stomach. There is, therefore, still plenty of time for the gastric acid to work on the starches during the remaining three or more hours that they are in the stomach before entering the small intestine. There, of course, the pancreatic juice completes the digestion of carbohydrate (starch, dextrin and the like), and also of protein, in a mainly alkaline medium.

Whether Dr Hay's explanation of his theory is right or wrong, however, does not really matter; the indisputable fact remains that his theory does most certainly work. As he pointed out, any professor of medicine who claims that it does not has never given it a fair trial, otherwise he could not with honesty make such a claim.

The Importance of the Chemical Balance

For optimum health and heightened resistance to disease the diet should, ideally, consist of alkali-forming foods and acid-forming foods in the ratio, approximately, of four to one, which, when metabolized, will produce a corresponding ratio in the body.

When Dr Hay was asked what was the scientific basis for this ratio, he replied: 'We have no way of arriving at the relative proportion of alkaline and acid elements needed by the body except through an analysis of its excretions. When we take into account all of the excretions through the four avenues of elimination, we find that the loss in alkali is four times as great as that in acid. This means that if we would replace our losses fully we need four times as much of the alkaline intake as of the acid intake. This is a fact well known to physiologists and can be verified in almost any work on physiology.'

With regard to the chemical balance of the human blood, Dr Hay wrote: 'It may seem strange that the slight difference between a pH 7.1 and 7.6 spells the wide difference between an acidosis and an alkalosis, yet this is true; and even this slight variation makes all the difference between function of the most chaotic variety and that of high efficiency.' Judging by the average of those of his patients who had conserved their alkaline reserve for several years through ob-serving the proper ratio of alkali-forming foods to acid-forming ones, the 'normal' alkalinity — as distinct from the 'average' one — should not be much below pH 7.5. From the standpoint of *averages* this is considered an alkalosis, yet when the alkalinity of the blood is sufficiently high to show a 7.5 pH, 'there is extremely high functional activity, with comparable feeling of good health, mental activity and physical efficiency.'

An interesting and important sidelight is thrown on this question of alkalinity by Dr Dudley d'Auvergne Wright in *Foods for Health and Healing* (Health Science Press, Sussex). He points out that 'the normal alkalin-ity of the body fluids is the most favourable one for the action of vitamins.'

It is not difficult to distinguish between alkali-forming and acid-forming foods:

Alkali-forming foods comprise all vegetables (including potatoes if cooked in their skins and the skins are eaten);* all salads; all fresh fruits (except plums and cranberries); almonds; milk.

Acid-forming foods comprise all animal proteins such as meat, fish, shell-fish, eggs, cheese, poultry; nuts

* In view of sprays that are used on potatoes today it is best to buy organically grown.

(except almonds); all the starch foods such as grains, bread and flour and other foods made from cereal starches; sugars.

Complete lists of both types of foods are given in the Appendix (page 254).

It should be emphasized at this point that there is sometimes confusion for some people regarding the classification of 'acid' fruits (grapefruit, oranges, lemons, berries, etc.) as 'alkali-forming'. It should therefore be understood that this classification does not relate to the 'acid' taste of the fruit but to its *end-product* in the body.* The acid fruits, moreover, are the foods which deposit the highest alkaline ash of all foods. It is an interesting fact that the acids of these fruits leave the body within an hour or so of being eaten. They do so via the lungs (mainly), and the skin, urinary tract and bowel. The alkalis, when released from their combination with the acids, provide a highly valuable contribution to the body's alkaline reserve. The only way in which acid fruits can be said to be 'acid-forming' is when they are wrongly combined with starches at the same meal, when they can cause an uncomfortable 'full-up' feeling, or even pain. The sufferer then concludes that acid fruits don't suit him!

In order to approximate the ideal four-to-one alkali-acid ratio the day's meals should include one protein meal only, one starch meal only, and one wholly alkaline meal, with occasionally two, or even three wholly alkali-forming meals. An occasional 'health day' on nothing but frequent meals of *one kind of fruit*

---

* It should also be emphasized with regard to the classification of concentrated starches and concentrated proteins as 'acid-forming', that this refers only to their end-products in the body, and *not* to the mediums necessary for their digestion, i.e. an *alkaline* medium for starches, and an *acid* medium for proteins.

— a *'gesundheitstag'* as it is called in Germany — is
highly beneficial. Young children and people doing
much manual work can, however, have extra starch
meals.

How to plan these meals is described in Part Two.

A word of warning is necessary here. To opt out of the
eating habits of the herd does require, at first, a certain
amount of self-discipline. For this reason compatible
eating is not recommended for people who are quite
content with their state of health, or who can eat
incompatible mixtures without discomfort or apparent
harm. Dr Hay warned that such people do not have the
very necessary 'burning desire' to recover from some
departure from health, or the will-power, 'guts' and
determination to see the thing through. He therefore
advised that any change in the diet should be made
slowly, by degrees. It was quite sufficient, to begin
with, he said, just to observe the starch-protein rule.
When this change is well established, the natural
wholefoods — especially those in uncooked, salad
form — should be gradually increased, and any refined
carbohydrates, and other processed foods, should be
proportionately decreased.

The number of alkali-forming meals should then be
increased. Especially recommended for beginners are
vegetable or salad meals containing delicious potato
dishes; they are not only less expensive but also more
satisfying in our cold climate than meals composed of
only vegetables, salads or fruit.

Compatible eating, it should be pointed out, can be
as cheap — or as expensive — as the housekeeping
purse dictates. And it is definitely more economical, as
small correctly-combined meals are better digested and
thus more satisfying than large orthodox meals; it is not
the amount of food that counts, but *the amount that is
properly digested, absorbed and metabolized by the body.*

Proof of this fact for followers of the Hay System is the falling-off of any desire for mid-morning snacks and afternoon tea with cakes and biscuits. In these days of soaring food prices *more nourishment for less food deserves serious consideration*.

It is important to note that observing the rules for compatible eating considerably reduces the amount of fat in the diet, especially those fats arbitrarily occurring in so many processed, supermarket foods today — and this reduction takes place despite the culinary use of cream which raises compatible eating to delicious heights of enjoyment. Cream, in moderation, is almost a necessity for this way of eating. *Healthwise*, there need be no cause for concern on this score as explained in Chapter Four. *Costwise*, the extra expense of cream is balanced by the reduction which compatible eating makes in other food costs, such as those of expensive, ready-made, 'instant' foods, and of the weekly meat bill. Apart from the starch-protein rule, the Hay System is in fact totally in line with the Royal College of Physicians' recent recommendations for a healthy diet.

It is even more important to note that observing the rules for compatible eating *automatically reduces* the acid-forming foods in the diet and *automatically increases* the alkali-forming foods rich in accessory food factors, thereby contributing to the alkaline reserve and a well-balanced body chemistry. In this correct chemical balance lies the secret of health and resistance to disease.

An interesting analogy, here, is provided by the fact that the correct alkali-acid balance is also of importance in the soil. In the *Soil Association Journal* of December 1973, Michael Blake draws attention to this fact and stresses that the effect of an imbalance is not restricted to the soil, but is of 'universal importance to all living organisms.'

Finally, it cannot be repeated too often that the Hay System is not a joyless, wearisome 'diet' but a 'philosophy of living'. A new convert, Joan Hodgson, enthusiastically agrees. In *A White Eagle Lodge Book of Health and Healing* (The White Eagle Publishing Trust, 1983) she writes: 'Harmonious food-combining is a way of life. Once the rules have become familiar, imaginative cooks can have fun thinking up the most delicious meals. This is not a régime of constant self-denial, but of rethinking the meals so that each one is based on family favourites with food combined in such a way that more nourishment can be extracted with less tax on the digestion, and consequently more energy for enjoying life.'

Fifty years of 'enjoying life' on the Hay System, and the experience gained in helping countless people to regain health by its means, have convinced me that health is our normal state, that we were designed, created, born to be healthy. This experience has also provided proof in plenty that correct eating can not only greatly improve the quality of life but can also prevent many of the degenerative diseases.

3.

THE HAY SYSTEM AND THE DEGENERATIVE DISEASES

The hope of humanity lies in the prevention of degenerative and mental diseases, not in the care of their symptoms.

Dr Alexis Carrel

There is a generally held belief today that people are living longer than formerly. Although more children survive to reach adult life, middle-aged people have scarcely improved upon the life-expectancy of their great-grandparents. The unpleasant truth is that, instead of living longer to a healthy and enjoyable old age, we are merely taking longer to die.

Moreover, with each generation there is an increase in the ordinary diseases of degeneration, and these are appearing at ever earlier ages than formerly. All the 'tremendous new discoveries' in the drug field have been unable to stem this increase. Belief in the curative power of drugs has contributed to this increase by diverting attention from the positive promotion of health.

As a result, the disillusioned drug-givers and drug-takers are now showing a healthy interest in the doctrine of 'holism' — treating the whole person rather than just the disease symptoms. This is completely in line with Dr Hay's commonsense principles, which more than ever before are shown to be valid. He advocated the treatment of the patient himself — not the symptoms — and argued that it was childish in the extreme to suppose we can restore a person to full health without first rooting out the cause of his disease;

to do otherwise was just as stupid as bailing out a leaky boat without first finding and stopping the leak.

Dr Hay also argued that this cause, in every case, is one and the same thing — *food* (over-consumption of refined carbohydrate, and incompatible combinations) — and pointed out that the degenerative diseases are just different manifestations of this one cause. The cure, he pointed out, 'therefore lies in food always and only.'

This *unitary conception of disease* bears a close resemblance to that advocated by Surgeon Capt. Cleave in *The Saccharine Disease* (except regarding incompatible combinations with which he was not in accord). He, too, indicts *food* (over-consumption of refined carbohydrate) as the cause of disease and he, too, points out that the degenerative diseases are just different manifestations of this one cause. This concept, known as 'the saccharine disease' (i.e., relating to sugar), is now grudgingly conceded by the medical establishment, and enthusiastically accepted by a growing number of doctors both here and abroad.

Among these manifestations Dr Cleave lists *constipation*, with its complications of varicose veins and haemorrhoids; *obesity; diabetes; skin diseases; dental decay* and *periodontal disease; urinary tract infections* (such as cystitis, from which so many women suffer today); and *coronary disease*. Dr Hay dealt with most of these manifestations and others as well, but nowhere in his many writings have I found any reference whatsoever to coronary heart disease (CHD).

This fact is highly significant; it confirms Dr Cleave's contention that it 'takes *time* for the consumption of refined carbohydrates to produce the various manifestations of the saccharine disease', and that these manifestations have 'incubating periods' which differ in each case. In the case of diabetes, for instance, the incubation period may be twenty years, but in the case of CHD, thirty years. As CHD was a rare disease from

1900 to 1930 when Dr Hay was practising medicine, it is not surprising that he never had to deal with it. It was still a rare disease in the 1920s and it was not until thirty years afterwards, in the 1950s, that CHD started to become an epidemic disease, *concurrent with the massively increasing consumption of refined sugar.*

CHD incidence in Britain is now among the highest in the world, and kills 170,000 people annually — one every three minutes — *and about 5,000 of these before the age of fifty.*

Doctors admit that what causes CHD is not known with any certainty, and that they are still ignorant of its dietary requirements. But on BBC-TV in June 1983, in a series of programmes called 'A Plague of Hearts', a new approach to preventing it was advocated by a leading epidemiologist, Professor Geoffrey Rose — the creation of *'a more healthy lifestyle for the whole population.'*

Dr Hay advocated this selfsame approach — not for CHD, which was virtually non-existent in his lifetime, but for treating and preventing *all* the degenerative diseases. There are a number of very good nutritional 'cures' now being promoted, but it can be stated categorically that the Hay System comes nearer to a full understanding of the causes, treatment, and prevention of disease than any other doctrine, as the following discussions of some of these degenerative diseases will confirm:

Constipation (Simple)
Fifty years ago William Howard Hay listed constipation as one of the main sources of acid formation in the system, and warned that, if long continued, it could be the cause of many of the degenerative diseases. Present-day medical findings have confirmed this warning and have also revealed that constipation is almost certainly a contributing factor to the high rate of bowel cancer in advanced nations.

Dr Hay also listed incompatible food combinations

and fibre-deficient refined carbohydrates as sources of acid formation. Both these sources directly contribute to constipation. Striking proof that they do so was provided in a paper entitled 'Amylaceous Dyspepsia' (starch-caused indigestion), published in *The Liverpool Medico-Chirurgical Journal* in 1931. Its author was Dr Lionel J. Picton, author-in-chief of the famous *Cheshire Medical Testament*, published in 1938, in which thirty-one family doctors declared that *the prevention of sickness depends on right feeding*.

In this paper Dr Picton drew attention to a well-known laboratory experiment on dogs by the famous Russian scientist, Pavlov. From this experiment, according to Dr Picton, Pavlov deduced the following data: minced beef fed to a dog is digested in about four hours, starch by itself passed through a dog's stomach in a much shorter time, in one-and-a-half hours or less, white bread more slowly than brown. *But when meat was mixed with the starch there was invariably a delay — a protracted delay*. Instead of four-and-a-half hours for meat alone, this mixture took eight or more hours to leave the stomach.

Dr Picton argued that this delay in one section of the line tended towards delay all along the line. As he pointed out: 'The somewhat startling conclusion flows from this, that meals of mixed character such as meat and bread favour constipation, whereas meat and salad at one meal and starchy food such as bread and butter at a separate meal have no such effect.'

Dr Picton's paper provided outstanding confirmation of the truth of the starch-protein concept, and of the close relationship of incompatible food mixtures to constipation. And his case histories of patients provided proof.

The first step in the treatment of constipation is therefore none other than that recommended by Dr Hay for all diseases, *the removal of the cause* — far too much acid-forming meat and carbohydrates (especially refined carbohydrates), far too little alkali-forming vegetables, salads and fruits, *and incompatible food mixtures*. Instructions for 'the removal of the cause' are given in Part Two; they are not difficult to follow and will soon prove to *simplify* meal-planning, and lessen cooking and the cost of cooking.

No matter how correctly the meals are combined, the fibre in the diet should always be increased by taking unprocessed wheat bran daily. It should be taken at first in teaspoonful doses, in water, before meals, increasing this gradually to suit individual needs. Neil S. Painter, well-known London surgeon, advises: 'You are eating enough bran only when you can pass soft stools without straining. Once you have found this amount take it for life.' Recent research has shown that in westernized countries the daily stool is hard and viscous compared to that of rural Africans and Asians living on unrefined foods, and that the intestinal transit time (the time taken for food to traverse the intestines) may be as long as *five days* instead of twenty-four hours. Thus many people who think that they are not constipated may be very constipated indeed, *despite having a daily stool*. For this reason, and in order to speed recovery from *any* disease, Dr Hay suggested taking a daily two-quart, cool, plain water enema, but not without professional instruction.

Indigestion
(Standard type — upper abdominal pain, heartburn, sometimes accompanied by acid regurgitation)
This is a condition which for many people has become an accepted evil and part of their lives. It is most frequently caused by treacherous food mixtures and it responds with astonishing rapidity to compatibly combined ones. I have rescued many people from afternoon indigestion pains resulting from lunchtime sandwiches of bread and cheese, or bread and meat. They all marvelled at the ensuing peace and tranquillity in their interiors!

Dr Cleave argues that the main cause of indigestion is the refining of carbohydrate foods which strips them of proteins so that there results an outpouring of gastric secretion but not enough protein to neutralize it.* This argument, however, is somewhat difficult to reconcile with the fact that, in spite of eating refined carbohydrate foods (white bread and sugar) during the whole of my first year of compatible eating, I nevertheless lost indigestion of fifteen years' duration during the very first week.

Dr Hay, too, was convinced that in many, perhaps most cases of indigestion, refined carbohydrates were the cause, but for a different reason. Dr Lionel Picton was likewise convinced. In the aforementioned paper he states that his evidence for this conviction was 'mainly clinical', having found that reduction of refined starchy food intake relieved his patients' symptoms. For 'the incipient dyspeptic' Dr Picton recommended 'a dietary in which more greens and grilled meat should replace some of the bad foods of modern times, and moreover a diet in which starchy foods should be separated as far as possible from meat, and taken at separate meals' — a 'dietary' totally in accord with Dr Hay's precepts.

Naturopath Harry Benjamin is another who believes that combinations of starch and protein foods can cause digestive trouble. In *Your Diet in Health and Disease* (Thorsons, 1974) he recommends cutting out bread and potatoes with meat.

Dr Hay warned that taking antacids, the patent 'cure' for indigestion, is not the answer; they can compound the trouble, leading to more serious conditions. There have been medical warnings today that antacids can use up certain vitamins in the body which are vitally necessary for its proper functioning. Moreover, experi-

* *Peptic Ulcer* (John Wright & Sons Ltd, Bristol, 1962), Chapter 4.

ments at Cornell University U.S.A., revealed that giving carbonate of soda and milk caused a form of kidney stones in laboratory animals. Antacids are merely a crutch which deals with *the symptom instead of the cause*. The best treatment for indigestion is compatible eating.

Arthritis
The cause and cure of arthritis, whether rheumatoid or osteoarthritis, has baffled the medical profession. Doctors frankly admit as much; they prescribe anti-inflammatory drugs and painkillers, and tell their patients they must learn to live with it. The side-effects of the painkillers, however, can be serious, even lethal, as the effects of the new 'wonder-drug' for arthritis, *Opren* — now withdrawn — have recently proved all too tragically. 'No drug to date has cured, or ever will cure, a true case of arthritis,' wrote Dr Hay.

There are many contributing causes of arthritis, such as injuries, abuse of the body, allergic reactions, infections, stress-exhausted adrenal glands, vitamin D deficiency, etc. But the end result of most of the underlying causes produces one common denominator — deranged body chemistry. A main cause is therefore an accumulation of acid end-products of digestion resulting in a lowered reserve of the alkaline buffer salts. Dr Hay stressed that 'the function of every organ and tissue depends on the height, breadth and depth of the alkaline reserve; and the lower this is the lower the function . . .'

The logical approach to treatment is therefore a nutritional one, aimed at the deranged body chemistry and *not at the joints* as in the conventional drug treatments and surgical treatments presently in vogue. These are merely palliatives which, once again, deal with the symptoms instead of grappling with the causes.

In a personal communication from Dr James Lambert

Mount [author of *Food and Health of Western Man* (Charles Knight & Co. Ltd, 1975), and one of the founders of the McCarrison Society] he described how he had successfully applied a nutritional approach when treating a hundred volunteer patients, suffering from arthritis, who took part in a trial in New Zealand. They were put on *a diet aimed at changing the body from an acid to an alkaline state*, by giving up red meat, flour, and sugar, and concentrating on salads, fruit and organ meats. There was an average eighty per cent success rate varying from considerable improvement in the arthritis to a complete cure.

Arthritis is considered the least amenable to treatment of all the chronic diseases. But Dr Hay maintained that arthritis responds to nutritional treatment as surely as do other degenerative diseases. Twenty-eight years of experience enabled him to write very positively — and comfortingly — about the ultimate cure of arthritis:

> Most cases of arthritis are curable, and permanently so, if the disease has not progressed to such a degree that it has permanently destroyed the function of the affected joint as occurs in ankylosis. As long as there is motion left in any joint, the case is by no means hopeless. Do not be discouraged if the pain seems to inhibit motion completely, if at the same time the joint can be moved passively to any degree.

He warned, however, that deposits outside the circulation, as those in the tissues about the joints, may require years to be completely absorbed or may never be fully absorbed, yet the joints become usable, and pliable, without pain. But he promised that even cases of severe arthritis, when every joint in the body is affected with pain and immobility, recover uniformly when the body is relieved of its excessive debris and feeding is corrected.

No specific diet is necessary, or even advisable, he said, for arthritis, but it is essential that the food intake should be largely of the alkali- or base-forming variety — vegetables, salads, fruits — and kept so throughout life; that the colon should be brought up to date and kept so. It is essential that the diet should contain fresh, properly constituted foods, whole foods, and *as much as possible of these in raw form*. It is interesting that, in 1936, at the Royal Free Hospital in London, an experiment on arthritic patients with a raw diet was successfully carried out by Dr Dorothy C. Hare. In the report of this experiment Dr Hare stressed the fact that the rawness of the food seemed to be the one outstanding factor that brought about results.*

Dr Hay warned that starches and sugar, carbohydrates of concentrated character, are the chief dietary causes of arthritis, not so much because they are so intrinsically causative, as because they are usually eaten in combination with incompatible foods and their proper digestion prevented, with resulting fermentation.

The elimination of starches and sugar in the diet is therefore of paramount importance. In the opinion of some authorities at the present time most arthritic patients experience difficulty in assimilating carbohydrates, with ensuing indigestion. (Once again, starch is the villain of the piece, and even a valuable wholegrain one can be so if not correctly combined with other foods.) From my own experience, and that of correspondents and friends, indigestion frequently precedes and accompanies arthritis. This indicates that both conditions are due to the same cause — incompatible food mixtures and a lowered alkaline reserve. This underlines the great value of compatible eating; it automatically reduces the amount of starch eaten and ensures its compatible combination with other foods.

Many of Dr Hay's patients recovered fully by making no other dietary change apart from the strict separation

---

* *Proceedings of the Royal Society of Medicine*, Vol 30, 1936.

of incompatible foods (as in my own case). But to make this strict separation, and at the same time to make the diet 80 per cent alkali forming, is more effective, speedier, and helps to correct the chemical balance. Arthritis, asserted Dr Hay, is a purely nutritional state, the result of an imbalance in the body's chemistry; he found this was evident from observation of many cases. He also found it evident that 'exposure to weather, or occupational pursuits, have nothing to do with the creation of the condition, except in a secondary way.'

To help correct the chemical balance and increase the delicate alkaline reserve in the blood-stream, Dr Hay particularly recommended a sufficiency of acid fruits such as oranges, grapefruit, and lemons (the juice of a lemon — now, alas, so expensive — in a glass of water on waking is very beneficial); these acid fruits are especially high in alkaline salts — lemons most of all. Unfortunately, many arthritic sufferers make the mistake of avoiding all 'acid fruits' thinking thereby to help their condition, whereas they are merely worsening an already deficient intake of vitamins. As there seems to be much confusion regarding the term 'acid fruits' the reader is urged to re-read its classification in Chapter Two.

Dr Hay also recommended:

● Celery juice; this has proved invaluable in dissolving and removing years of accumulated acid deposits in the cartilage of arthritic joints. In *The Home Herbal* (Pan Paperback), Barbara Griggs recommended celery seeds for arthritis and rheumatism because their 'high alkaline value helps to counteract acid formation in the blood and clear it out of the system.' Arthritis sufferers will find her other recommendations most helpful.

● Wheatgerm, bran, kelp (seaweed, obtainable in tablet form at health food shops), and *cod liver oil*. Dr

Hay claimed that that these supplements are also very beneficial for *all* departures from health.

- *Gentle exercise, rest*, and *natural sunlight*. Research by Dr John Ott, famous pioneer of time-lapse photography, confirmed the great benefit to arthritis of natural sunlight. In *Health and Light* (The Devin Adair Co., Conn., U.S.A.) he proved with regard to his own arthritis that spending as much time as possible out of doors, walking or gardening, and receiving natural sunlight energy (even on dull days) directly through the eyes, *minus sunglasses, spectacles, or contact lenses*, is highly beneficial in the control of this disease.

- The elimination from the diet of *vinegar, spices, tea, coffee* and *alcohol* — especially sweet wines and liqueurs.

- *Calmness and emotional control*; tension, fear, anger, hate, etc. do much to aggravate arthritis symptoms and increase suffering.

It must therefore be repeated again: *arthritis is a purely nutritional state and its logical treatment is a nutritional one*. Unfortunately arthritis research foundations have been issuing statements for many years that nutritional therapy is totally without merit, thus discouraging most doctors from paying attention to their patients' diet. Any cure or improvement resulting from nutritional therapy has therefore been dismissed as a 'spontaneous remission'. There is now, however, too much solid evidence of sustained benefit from such therapy to justify this concept. Such a remission, of course, does occur.

Obesity
This is a far more serious condition than most people

realize; it is now closely linked with diabetes, cholesterol-rich gallstones and coronary artery disease. Roughly half the people in this country are overweight, and obesity among children is now reaching epidemic proportions.

It is generally believed that people become obese because they eat too much. Dr Hay believed that obesity is far more often evidence of an imbalance in nutrition than the result of eating too much, and that its cause lies very frequently in the mixture of starch food and proteins, or starches with acid fruits. He also strongly indicted refined carbohydrates, as did Dr T.L. Cleave fifty years later.

The logical treatment of obesity, therefore, whether this is of slight or severe degree, is to correct the faulty eating habits that led up to this condition. Compatible eating is especially effective. According to many reports I have received from Hay System followers, *merely avoiding warring mixtures is sufficient gradually to reduce excess weight — without even trying to do so; without feeling hungry; without wearisome calorie counting; and without resorting to crash slimming diets, appetite-suppressors and dangerous fat-reducing drugs*. Dr Hay warned that all so-called fat-reducing remedies 'should be avoided as you would the plague', as they are a snare and a delusion, and their very slight results are paid for at a fearful cost in vitality and health. His warning has now received ample confirmation in a report by the consumer magazine *Which?* of 13 April 1983; it had harsh words for certain quick-slimming products which not only fail in their objective but also have unpleasant side-effects.

Attempts to lose weight quickly are not recommended. Any change in the diet should be made gradually. To start losing weight it is therefore sufficient just to become accustomed to separating the incompatible classes of foods into different meals. When this separation is well established, the number of alkali-forming meals should be increased. An excellent and easy way of doing this (if desired) is to make breakfast consist solely of fruit, or fruit and yogurt, making the fruit one kind of fruit only. Doing so will cause no drop in energy for the day's work — *the energy for today is provided by the foods eaten yesterday;* eating a large breakfast actually ties up some of one's energy during the morning. Dr Hay always counselled that 'the best breakfast of all is no breakfast at all'! — but not if eating orthodox meals.

Many people are not at all hungry for breakfast, but sheer habit forces them to eat. Dr Hay always taught: '*never eat anything of any kind at any time unless you feel really hungry . . .* you will get far more nourishment out of foods that are eaten when you are very hungry than if these same foods are eaten without proper hunger.' This excellent rule is not only of importance for slimmers but also for everyone who is health conscious. Dr Cleave considered it of such importance that he listed it as rule number one in his Natural Diet for Health (*The Saccharine Disease,* page 188): '*Do not eat any food unless you definitely want it.*' It is a fact that most of us eat far more food than we need. There is truth in the saying that 'we live on a third of the food we eat — the doctor lives on the other two-thirds!'

There is no need to go without any good, unprocessed, unrefined, whole food while reducing weight, provided that it is eaten compatibly. Even the so-called fattening foods, bread and potatoes, can be eaten with impunity, provided that the bread is wholewheat bread (preferably home-baked — see Part Four), the potatoes are cooked in their skins and the skins eaten, and care is taken not to 'plaster' both the bread and potatoes with too much butter. Fats should be used with care by slimmers, especially in the form of full-fat cheeses; the cottage cheeses are best, as long as they contain no added salt. The intake of salt should be drastically reduced in the diet of slimmers (and considerably reduced in the diet of most people).

Obesity is closely associated with constipation, indigestion, and arthritis. The advice that is good for the
treatment of these conditions is therefore good for the
treatment of obesity: the removal of the cause — refined
carbohydrates — especially all sugars and *hidden* sugars
— and incompatible food mixtures; ensuring that the
bulk of the food intake consists of the alkali-forming
fresh vegetables, salads and fruits; eliminating foods
not recommended; eating as much food as possible in
raw form; keeping the colon up to date by every
possible means; and not forgetting the daily ration of
fresh, unprocessed bran, and other food supplements.

With regard to exercise — the time-worn remedy for
excessive deposits of fat — Dr Hay warned that forced
exercise should never be taken in order to slim: 'burning up the fats through exercise increases one's appetite
tremendously and consequently the total of foods of all
kinds consumed'. Exercise while slimming should be of
the moderate kind.

Paradoxically, compatible eating is equally helpful to
people who are under-weight! Both conditions are due
to abnormal states of body chemistry. Therefore, just as
compatible eating produces a steady loss of weight for
those who are overweight, so will it also produce a
gradual building up of weight for those who are too
thin — the only difference being that thin people can
make more use of the starch foods. Thin people should
be warned, however, that they, too, will lose weight *at
first*. This is no cause for concern and is merely an
adjustment, 'a throwing off of the old in preparation for
the building of the new.'

The Hay System is first and foremost a normalizing régime.
This fact clearly indicates that nature works continually
to restore us to the ideal in weight, stature, health,
efficiency and everything else, when we remove the
obstacles in the way of her remarkable healing power.

Diabetes Mellitus

Of the two kinds, 'late onset diabetes' and 'early onset diabetes', Dr Hay's writings concerned the former; the latter was rare in his time as children in the early 1900s did not consume fibre-deficient junk food as they do today.

There are over 600,000 diabetics in Britain. For twenty years their doctors have been advising them to cut down drastically on carbohydrate foods and eat a high fat diet. But, in November 1982, British doctors admitted that they have been on the wrong track and for twenty years have been giving the wrong advice to their diabetic patients.

Dietary Recommendations for Diabetics for the 1980s — A Policy Statement by the British Diabetic Association, published in 1982, has turned the conventional diet on its head, 'because of its potential cardiovascular risks.' Instead of the traditional low-carbohydrate, high-fat diet, this Policy Statement now recommends a diet containing much less fat but *a high proportion of unrefined carbohydrate foods* — a remarkable tribute to the dietary concepts of Surgeon Capt. Cleave which, till the 1970s, were derided by his fellow physicians.

The Policy Statement also recommends the avoidance of all sugar and emphasizes the value of fresh fruits and vegetables.

The B.D.A.'s new dietary recommendations provide striking confirmation and vindication of Dr Hay's own beliefs and dietary recommendations at the beginning of the century; he, too, was convinced that he and his medical colleagues had been giving 'the wrong advice'; he, too, advocated a diet containing a high proportion of unrefined 'fibrous carbohydrate foods' instead of the traditional low-carbohydrate diet; and he, too, recommended strict moderation in fat intake and emphasized the value of plenty of fresh fruit and vegetables.

His dietary recommendations for diabetes, moreover, were enunciated, *seventy-one years before the pub-*

lication of the B.D.A.'s Policy Statement in 1982, in a paper read before the United States Warren County Medical Society in 1911.

In this paper on diabetes mellitus Dr Hay stated: 'The very men and women whose daily food comes most nearly up to the standard of diet prescribed for diabetics are the men and women in whom the cases of diabetes are most numerous and most fatal. They are the people whose daily ration is filled with fish, flesh and fowl, and in which but little room is left for bread and potatoes.'

This paper is thought to be the very first piece of written material dealing with the Hay System. It was lost for nearly thirty years, but soon after Dr Hay's death in 1940 it was fortunately found by the purchaser of his old desk, jammed with other papers behind one of its drawers. It is of special value and significance for Dr Hay's followers; it revealed that *he was having remarkable success in restoring former late onset diabetics to health, without drugs, eleven years before Banting and Best discovered insulin*. He did so by telling his patients 'to quit the meat, eggs and fish which had formed the principal part of their nourishment for so long and to eat a baked potato once a day, a slice of toasted whole-wheat bread and all the juicy fruits that were desired' (he had not at this stage developed the starch-protein concept). The improvement on this régime, he affirmed, 'was marked and very gratifying to the patient, not only because of an increase in strength but in appetite and spirits and, what seemed at first strange, there never was a marked increase in the amount of sugar voided and this was even diminished . . .' (He also instructed his patients to keep their elimination up to date by every possible means, including daily two-quart enemas of cool, plain water.)

Dr Hay's success in treating diabetics in this way convinced him completely that a strict adherence to his plan for long enough would result in complete cure of all those cases in which there was no grave organic change. But to the medical pundits at that time his treatment for diabetics was rank blasphemy. For one thing, diabetes had always been considered incurable; for another thing, all avenues of relief had been explored without success. *Yet here was a man who preached that diabetes was curable without the use of drugs.* So they branded him a charlatan and ostracized him — they could do no less to safeguard their professional integrity.

Dr Hay, dismissed as a 'charlatan', was in truth an unrecognized and humble genius who had found the key, not only to diabetes mellitus, but to all the degenerative diseases.

Allergy

'Allergy,' wrote Dr Hay, 'is a specific lack of body resistance to certain irritants whether of food, pollens, foreign proteins or whatever,' but, he affirmed, *'the cause lies in the individual and not in the environment.'* The irritants are merely the secondary cause (irritants, here, meaning naturally-occurring ones, not man-created environmental poisons in food, air, and water, to which the healthiest body has little resistance); the primary cause being almost wholly in what we eat and how we eat it, and in a disturbed state of the body chemistry. He promised that a hay fever sufferer can so change his body chemistry 'that he can bury his face in his former *bête noir,* no matter what this happens to be, without a single sneeze.'

During the past few decades very strong support for Dr Hay's concept, linking allergies to disturbed body chemistry, has come to light through the work of Dr John Ott. In his book, *My Ivory Cellar* (Twentieth Century Press Inc., 1958) he describes a project to determine the action of ragweed pollen grains. While working on this project he produced visible evidence that the primary cause of hay fever may well be this disturbed body chemistry and not the contact with the pollen grain as universally believed. Time-lapse microscopic photography revealed that grains of ragweed pollen placed in nasal secretion from hay fever sufferers immediately started to emit tiny droplets of liquid. These droplets did not form, however, when ragweed pollen grains were placed in nasal secretions from persons not subject to hay fever.

Dr John Ott surmized from this that the body chemistry of hay fever sufferers was exactly right to make the ragweed pollen grains give off the droplets of fluid and that these could possibly be the factor which irritated the nasal membranes and not the mere contact with the outer surface of the pollen grains themselves. He suggests that if this is so, hay fever could then be prevented by altering the patient's chemical balance instead of trying merely to alleviate the trouble with medicines after the hay fever has once set in — a typical example of shutting the stable door after the horse has bolted!

Compatible eating acts as a double protection against allergy: as well as greatly improving the chemical balance (it takes about five years of correct eating to achieve — or approximate — the ideal state) it also ensures against the allergy-causing potential of incompletely digested proteins (see Chapter Two).

It is well known that, when proteins are incompletely broken down, imperfectly digested, they split up into intermediate or large protein molecules that are actually toxic, instead of into amino acids, their proper end-products. Some of these protein molecules constitute the substance known as histamine, well-known to medical specialists as a toxic protein which can be responsible for many common allergies such as hay fever, asthma, migraine, eczema, and urticaria. The liver of a healthy person can quickly destroy histamine whereas a damaged liver cannot.

Dr Daniel Munro relates, in *Man Alive, You're Half*

Dead!, how he found an excellent way of testing his allergic patients for the toxic proteins created by the mixed meal. He used on them a histamine-destroying substance, histaminase, and by so doing was able to discover 'with a considerable degree of accuracy' to what extent the mixed meal produces toxic end-products. He found that these patients required more units of histaminase to control their symptoms when eating mixed meals than when eating correctly combined ones — proof that the mixed meal produces more histamine. Dr Munro considered that this evidence alone was sufficient to justify compatible food combinations. When his patients were taught to avoid bad combinations many lost their symptoms entirely. (As one of the many benefits of natural yogurt, not sugared and flavoured, is its ability to inhibit the production of histamine, allergy sufferers might experience some relief from symptoms by eating daily a sufficiency of this natural antihistamine — so much safer than the toxic drug form.)

A report of an allergy conference in *Hospital Doctor* of 6 August 1981 revealed that the management of the allergic patient in Britain is worse than for almost any other disease. The usual treatment is suppression of the allergy symptoms by means of drugs and aerosols — treatment which deals only with the *manifestation* of the cause and not the fundamental cause itself: the patient's eating habits and (increasingly) chemical pollutants in his environment. Pioneers in the new discipline of clinical ecology, like Dr Mackarness, who are tackling the fundamental causes of allergy, are having spectacular results especially in those cases where suspect food additives have been producing hyperkinesis (over-activity) and serious behavioural problems in children. Needless to say, the concepts of these researchers in clinical ecology are challenging orthodox medical thinking and arousing the same medical disbelief and rejection as did the nutritional concepts of Dr Hay.

The results of these pioneers, however, would be even more spectacular if they taught their patients how to improve their body chemistry by adopting compatible eating; these patients would then be able within two or three months to restore to their diet all health-giving natural foods to which they were formerly allergic, and as Dr Hay promised, they would soon be able to bury their faces in their former *bête noir*, whether this be pollen, house dust, animal fur, synthetics or whatever, 'without a single sneeze'.

It was encouraging to find, while doing research for this book that, in the 1930s, at least one doctor in Britain agreed with Dr Hay that warring mixtures are detrimental to allergy sufferers. In *The Treatment of Asthma* (H.K. Lewis & Co. Ltd, 1936) Dr Harrington warns that mixtures of acid fruits, such as grapefruit, and starches, should be avoided at the same meal, and that acid fruits taken with large quantities of bread and butter are especially bad for asthma sufferers.

Skin Diseases
Being visible, skin diseases are a valuable indication of the state of health of the whole body. Their cause, as with all other diseases, is traceable to a toxic state of the body. The disease itself is evidence of the body throwing off toxic debris by passing it through the skin.

Why, in some people, should it be passed through the skin? The answer is that toxic debris finds an outlet through many different manifestations of the degenerative diseases, the particular form taken being determined by the specific resistance of the various organs. 'Here', wrote Dr Hay, 'is where heredity comes in. The *form* of disease is determined largely by the inheritance, but the *fact* of disease is determined by the individual.' It is therefore the weakest link in the hereditary chain which determines the organ, tissue or function to give way first.

After nearly thirty years of applying the principles of

natural treatment of disease, Dr Hay affirmed that he had seen no case of psoriasis or eczema that did not disappear after a few weeks or a very few months of separation of the incompatible foods, even though both conditions failed to improve under the most scientific treatment of many prominent skin specialists. And he urged: 'Treat all skin eruptions as external evidences of internal intoxication. Set about correcting all the causes of intoxication at once, and watch the results.' These results, being on the outside of the body, can provide an excellent visible demonstration of the Hay System at work, and of its astonishing efficacy when faithfully carried out.

Much of this internal intoxication — Dr Hay bluntly referred to it as 'internal filth' — arises from the fermentation and putrefaction of incompletely digested carbohydrate. Once again, the troublemakers are sugar and white flour foods — but especially sugar where skin diseases are concerned. In *The Saccharine Disease*, Dr Cleave confirms this fact: 'The relationship of many cases of eczema, especially in children, to the consumption of sugar, sweets and confectionery is well known, and in the author's opinion chronic furunculosis is the surest sign of high sugar consumption *and is most quickly arrested by stopping it.'*

Some years ago I witnessed a remarkable demonstration of this fact in the case of a ten-year-old boy who had had eczema since birth. He had been to specialist after specialist but was getting worse instead of better. At the age of ten his eczema was so bad that his classmates shunned any contact with him, and the members of his family were being kept awake at night with his moanings and scratchings. When his mother, in despair, brought him to see me, his arms and legs were a solid weeping mass of eruptions. I instructed her to cut out all his sugary breakfast cereals, his colas and fizzy 'pop' drinks, sweets, cakes and biscuits, and to substitute fresh fruit for puddings at his main meal.

I also instructed his mother how to make her own 'no-kneading', wholewheat bread. Ten days later she rang to tell me that *the eczema had vanished*, that nothing remained but shadows where the weeping eruptions had been. I was totally astonished at the speed of this boy's recovery — *in ten days after ten years of misery and the total failure of orthodox treatment*! His mother said her son had been most co-operative, was enjoying his new diet — especially the home-baked bread! — and was 'thrilled to bits' to have normal healthy skin for the first time in his life. Significantly, no skin specialist consulted had ever mentioned 'diet'.

The first thing to do in the treatment of eczema and other skin diseases, therefore, is to eliminate all sugar and sugar-containing foods from the diet; the sugar acts by providing the right condition in the gut to favour the proliferation of harmful products. When these are absorbed into the blood-stream, they can be responsible for acne, chronic boils, eczema, and many other skin conditions.

The second thing to do is to restore the body, as far as possible, to the proper chemical balance by adopting compatible eating.

Lastly, beauty-conscious women will be delighted to know that compatible eating does more than cure skin diseases; it also ensures a beautiful and flawless complexion. In *The Joy of Beauty* (Century Publishing, London, 1983) Leslie Kenton affirms that the vital acid-alkaline balance is an important aspect of any diet for 'super' health and beauty and one that most nutritional systems completely overlook. 'For we can reach truly positive health — health beyond the simple absence of disease — and remain permanently healthy only when the foods we eat supply us with a surplus of alkali-reacting foods.'

The Common Cold

'Colds are not caught; they are created with the feet under the

dinner table, and in no other way.' This was Dr Hay's commonsensical belief.

The common belief, however, is that colds are created through catching a cold germ — it is so much easier to look for the cause in a germ than in our wrong living habits. But the *primary* cause of colds is not the cold germ but the state of the chemistry of the body that provides a suitable soil for the proliferation of this type of germ. Moreover, if the cold germ were the primary cause of the common cold, then everybody, everywhere, would be having colds all the time. This is not the case, however, despite the fact that the germs found in the excretions from the nose and throat during colds are the selfsame, ubiquitous germs found anywhere at any time.

It is therefore evident that something protects the ones who escape infection, and this is the very thing that determines the cause of colds. As Dr Hay pointed out, 'Individual susceptibility or immunity is determined by each individual's condition at the time, and if you are cultivating an internal condition that makes for susceptibility then you may look for frequent colds when these are epidemic, or you can look for complete immunity during even the extreme peak of epidemic colds or influenza.' Hay System adherents have proved the truth of this statement and found themselves virtually immune from colds, as I myself have done — my record being twenty years without so much as a sniffle.

Although much time-and-money-consuming research during the past fifty years has been directed at finding the causes and cure of the common cold, medical science admits that these are still a mystery. Knowing the causes, Dr Hay understandably questioned 'what particular brand of stupidity could ever have made such research seemingly necessary in the first place?' He warned that no progress would ever be made until 'the germ theory' was dropped and the fact accepted that *every cold is merely an expression of the body's effort to clean house*. If the cold is evidence of the body's effort to get rid of objectionable waste material that is hampering its normal functioning, then its prevention lies in the elimination of this hampering waste. But the usual treatment is not directed towards this elimination but to fussing with end results, to soothing the mucous membranes involved with sedative or antiseptic inhalents, cough remedies or gargles. These remedies are directed towards *symptoms*, and not one is directed towards the removal of *the causes* that alone can produce the disagreeable and sometimes dangerous symptoms that we call a cold.

Nature herself indicates how to set about removing the causes by the fevers and loss of appetite which often accompany a severe cold. Therefore the best possible thing to do is to cut out all meals and do a fruit juice fast or, preferably, a fruit fast. The saying 'feed a cold and starve a fever' is badly misinterpreted. It really means that if you feed a cold you will end up having to starve a fever. The fruit fast is very pleasant; as much of any one kind of fruit desired every two hours throughout the day, for several days or even a week. Each day a different fruit can be chosen.

There is, however, a speedy way of breaking up a cold, but it involves much self-discipline and should not be undertaken unless with the approval and advice of the family doctor or a qualified naturopath. It involves taking a hot bath at night, as hot as one can stand; sipping a quart of hot water and lemon juice while in the bath; staying in the bath till sweating freely; then wrapping up in a blanket and lying under heavy covers to continue the sweat as long as possible; taking a purge in the morning on an empty stomach and eating no food till late afternoon, the first meal then consisting of fruit and vegetables before returning to a normal régime. An effective but somewhat drastic remedy for a cold!

It is far better to live so that colds cannot develop; the day is fast approaching when we will be as ashamed to admit to a cold as to a term in prison. 'But if you have sinned and a cold is the penalty', wrote Dr Hay, 'clean house just as nature would do through a longer time, but do it first!'

Headaches

A headache is one of the commonest afflictions that plague us, especially among women.

It is generally believed that not much can be done for it, and heredity usually gets the blame, particularly if mother and grandmother have both been sufferers. Like every other disease, heredity largely determines the form, as specific reistances are inherited, but as Dr Hay has pointed out over and over again, 'Like disease of every other sort, headaches cannot be inherited but must be created by the individual.'

Apart from those headaches caused by sunstroke, or pressure on the cervical nerves by displacement of the vertebrae, every case of headache marks a toxic state. In the case of migraine, for instance, each attack marks the end-point of the body's toleration for the toxins that have caused the trouble. A migraine attack is nature's effort to unload these toxins so that the body can be restored to a less toxic state and its function improved to normal; hence the sickness, the vomiting (frequently) and loss of appetite. Most migraine sufferers report feeling better for a time after each attack.

This improved state would continue for the sufferer and there would be no more migraines if the causes were not repeated. But the causes *are* repeated and the whole vicious circle starts over and over again.

One of Dr Hay's hundreds of successful cases is worth relating; this one being a pure case of serendipity. A woman of eighty-three asked to see him before a lecture in a college town as she had something very interesting to tell him. Her son had consulted Dr

Hay three months previously for indigestion, and had been directed to combine his foods compatibly. She thought it would make it easier for her son to keep to his new régime if she followed it also. To her immense astonishment, *within the first week* of doing so she lost a continuous and often severe headache that had plagued her every day of her life since she was fifteen years old — *that is, for sixty-eight years*! and she had made no other change in her eating habits apart from combining her foods compatibly.

As well as eating compatibly, however, Dr Hay advised 'bringing the colon up to date and keeping it up to date' by means of thorough enemas, 'for it is in the colon that so much starchy fermentation occurs due to the delay in discharging the unsplit starches found there.' This means alone, he affirmed, would cure a very large percentage of headaches. But in order to complete the guarantee of permanent relief it was necessary to separate foods into compatible groups. 'Any headache that persists in spite of this could be safely set down to pressure on the cranial nerves as they emit from the neck and can be taken care of perfectly by the osteopath or the chiropractor.'

Headache is really a very simple thing to understand and to treat when considered from the standpoint of the cause — a toxic state of the body. When this self-created cause has been removed, the body itself makes the cure.

Dental Decay
To Dr Hay toothache was merely an evidence of wrong chemical conditions of the body.

He affirmed that accumulation of the acid end-products of digestion and metabolism, or deficiencies in the normal alkaline reserve, is the entire cause not only of dental decay but also of all forms of inflammation of the gums and the entire category of mouth diseases.

No amount of cleanliness or meticulous hygiene of the mouth, he wrote, would have any effect on these disagreeable conditions if the food lacked the necessary elements for any length of time. The first evidences of trouble are red marginal gums, later shrinking or receding; the furred or fissured or indented tongue, or the enlarged 'papillae' so commonly seen on the tip of the average tongue; the early decay of the teeth; and crowding of the arch with the teeth out of line and the bite interfered with. Dr Hay insisted that before any dentist is allowed to practise his teachers should assure themselves that he knows the meaning of these evidences and how to meet the conditions.

The dentists, however, have paid almost no attention to wrong diet as a cause of these conditions. Since the end of the last century they have been wholly concerned with the so-called 'Acid Theory' which states that caries is caused by 'bacteria in acid fermentation' (bacteria producing corrosive acid by fermenting sugar and other refined carbohydrate) — the so-called 'plaque'. The Acid Theory has therefore focused research on attacks on the teeth from *without* and obscured the increasingly accepted fact that decay *primarily* starts from *within*, in the dentine below the enamel. This theory accounts for the truth that despite their brilliant advances in dental technology, dentists are still no nearer solving the problem of dental decay. It also accounts for the dental profession's naively eager acceptance of the fluoridation of water-supplies as 'a key measure' towards solving the problem, and for mistakenly dignifying it as 'preventive medicine'.

Such acceptance reveals a lamentable sweeping-aside of the fundamental cause of dental decay — the present-day enormous consumption of sugar, sweets and other sugary carbohydrates. It also betrays a total ignorance of what preventive medicine is all about. In promoting this nostrum for dental decay dentists are merely treating *the sympton* — caries — instead of grappling with *the cause* — faulty nutrition. As Dr Carstairs pointed out in a BBC Reith lecture: 'To allay the symptom while failing to explore and, if possible, eradicate the cause has always been bad medicine.'

Dr Hay would have called fluoridation an outstanding example of 'bad medicine'; he continually emphasized the foolishness of trying to cure any condition without first removing the cause.

The dentists know very well that sugar is the chief cause of dental decay, but *always and only as it affects the teeth from without*. Thus they continually overlook the fact — well known to Dr Hay sixty years ago, and revealed by recent medical findings — *that sugar not only wreaks havoc on the teeth but also on the body as a whole*, and is now known to be responsible for many of the crippling degenerative diseases such as those discussed in this chapter, and the present, killing degenerative diseases — coronary heart disease and cancer of the colon.

In *The Lancet* of 5 February 1983 (page 282, 'Sugars and Dental Decay'), Dr Aubrey Sheiham, Department of Community Health, The London Hospital Medical School, states unequivocally: 'Sugar is the principal cause of the most common disease in industrialized countries.' He gives some excellent advice on how the sugar intake should be reduced, but always in the context of its direct action on the tooth surfaces. Nowhere does he point out sugar's close link with the degenerative diseases, or recommend a diet that would ensure resistance to caries attack from within the tooth. But he does state that dental caries is preventable and that 'enough is known about its prevention to mount a successful attack upon it.'

No successful attack has yet been mounted. Dental advice about sugar reduction is generally 'perfunctory', frequently soft-pedalled, and even promotes the belief that general nutrition *has nothing to do with making teeth more resistant to decay* — as in the Health Education

Council's policy document, *The Scientific Basis of Dental Health Education*.

One dentist and his wife, Richard and Elizabeth Cook, wholeheartedly disagree with this outrageous belief. In their book *Sugar Off!* (Great Ouse Press, 1983) they outline an excellent do-it-yourself nutritional method of maintaining one's own dental health which virtually eliminates all sugars and sugar-containing foods and drinks. (Although they do occasionally resort to sugar substitutes.) Having come to the conclusion that dental health was too valuable a property to be left in the exclusive control of dentists who are 'trained to mend and pull teeth, not to advise on dietetics', this husband and wife team decided to go it alone with this book; they firmly believe that 'no dentist can bestow or dispense dental health. This you have to get for yourself.' — *advice completely in line with Dr Hay's concepts*.

Even more in line with Dr Hay's somewhat revolutionary concepts, however, was the advice being propounded by a doctor-dentist, Martha Jones, in the 1930s. According to a report of her work in *The New York Sun* of 5 December 1934, *'the gist of her theory is that good teeth depend on the degree of alkalinity in the diet, that unless the diet contains more alkalines than acids, decay is likely to occur.'* For every serving of meat, or egg, or bread (all of which are acid-forming in their end-products), Dr Jones advised two servings of fruit and vegetables. And the things she said make a diet alkaline are root vegetables such as turnips, sweet potatoes etc.; leafy vegetables; fruits; most alkaline are the leafy vegetables and the thinner and greener the leaf the better. Dr Jones also taught that the diets of expectant mothers are all-important to the development of the teeth, and that the child's teeth will be strong and healthy *if the mother has a very alkaline diet*.

According to *Dental Products Report*, April 1975, *'Dietary control* of cavities and gum disease may soon replace the tooth brush and dental floss as the mainstay of a healthy mouth.' At the 110th midwinter meeting of the Chicago Dental Society, Dr H.A. Huggins of Colorado Springs reported that tailoring diets to the needs of individual patients had produced remarkably good results where brushing and flossing had failed. Moreover, blood sample studies from more than 7,000 people and trace mineral analysis of their hair had led to the conclusion that *dental disease is actually a whole body disease*. This conclusion is totally in accord with that of Dr Hay and of Dr T.L. Cleave, with regard to dental disease.

It appears from the following remarkable case history described by Dr Hay that a correct diet can not only *prevent* dental decay but also *regenerate* cavities. He told how a young man had suffered from a row of cavities at the gum level that nearly encircled his upper and lower teeth. These were so sensitive to hot and cold, sweet and sour, that he was living largely on gruels and mushes; his dentist had insisted that it was useless doing anything for his cavities. At this time the young man came across the Hay System and determined to give it a trial. After six months he visited his dentist who perceived no change in his mouth. Six months later, however, he found his teeth were no longer sensitive and he was able again to chew hard foods with comfort. When his dentist examined his teeth again he was so astounded at what he saw that he collected a gathering of dentists to see this unusual case. 'Every cavity was now the seat of small deposits of secondary dentine — nature's effort at repairs — a scar tissue exactly suited to repair of the tissues of the teeth. This secondary dentine was as hard as the original enamel, as his dentist proved on testing it with a drill. As a result he kept all his teeth, and reported that he was happier and healthier than he had ever been in his life of well over forty years, never tiring, or running into depressed states, but always cheerful and optimistic.'

As far as dental decay is concerned, orthodox treatment has been unable to prevent it. Fluoridation has failed — the world-wide recent decline in dental decay in children is not related to either naturally occurring or artificial fluoridation — and there is evidence *which has never been disproved* that the latter is causing harm ranging from dental fluorosis in children (the first sign of poisoning from too much fluoride) to skeletal fluorosis in the elderly. Dr Hay counselled: 'Take care of the whole man and the teeth will take care of themselves, with or without a toothbrush.'

Postscript
Lack of space prevents further discussion of degenerative diseases in the context of compatible eating. But those discussed above are sufficient to confirm Dr Hay's contention (and that of Dr Cleave) that all degenerative disease has the same cause, no matter what its myriad manifestations; that its fundamental cause is improper diet and its cure 'lies in food always and only.'

Alas, there are a few degenerative diseases that do not respond to correct nutrition. One of these is 'Paralysis Agitans'. 'This', wrote Dr Hay, 'is the so-called Parkinson's Disease, a degenerative change in the nerves, supposedly in the centres of the sympathetic flexi. The condition is incurable by any means known so far, though many theories have been advanced and many remedies tried. It is a lamentable fact that when nerves of either sensation or motion begin to die, it is impossible to do anything constructive-looking toward a cure.' (Toward amelioration, yes — new drugs have helped considerably.)

Cancer — the second highest cause of death among adults in the Western nations, now killing more children than any other illness and the most dreaded of all degenerative diseases — is another condition for which virtually nothing has been done to 'cure'. In *The New Ecologist* of November/December 1978, in his article

'The National Cancer Institute and the fifty-year cover up', Peter Barry Chowka quoted the following statement of Dr William Howard Hay, published in *Cancer Journal*, 1927:

> Think back over the years of cancer research, of the millions spent, the time consumed, the pains expended . . . and where are we still today? Isn't it time to take stock of our basic concept to see if there isn't something radically wrong to account for the years of utter and complete failure to date? . . . Cancer has been consistently on the increase . . . *Is it possible that the cause of cancer is our departure from natural foods?*

In this same article, Mr Chowka explains how, fifty years ago, encouraging leads established a clear relationship between diet and cancer, but focus by cancer establishments on symptomatic treatment rather than on prevention had virtually covered up the real answer to prevention and cure of cancer, '*the return to a healthy diet.*'

Now, at long last, this close relationship between diet and cancer is again being recognized — seventy years after Dr Hay had shown the way. There are now increasing medical reports that thirty per cent, or even fifty per cent, of all cancer cases are the result of 'unhealthy lifestyles' and *improper diet. Hospital Doctor* of 16 June 1983 reported that at a meeting of the Imperial Cancer Research Fund in London on 13 June, a change in lifestyle and diet was suggested by Sir Richard Doll as 'the key to cancer cure': 'Stop smoking, drink less alcohol, become slim and eat more fibre and vegetables and less animal fat and fatty dairy products.'

Dr Hay said truly when he wrote: 'Verily, we are dunces when it comes to our treatment of our own bodies, for we are misinterpreting nature's plainest warnings and trying to avoid even seeing them, covering them up with the action of so-called remedies instead of removing the whole foolish condition.'

The truth is that we have fed our animals with far more intelligence than we have fed ourselves. The stockman has always recognized that when his domestic animals were fed correctly they remained well, and when fed wrongly they fell sick. It is worthy of note, here, and of particular significance to the argument of this present book, that even the canine species benefits from compatible eating! The famous vet, 'Buster' Lloyd-Jones, warned dog owners in *Love on a Lead*: 'Don't mix biscuits with meat or gravies. It can cause digestive disturbance.'

It is very encouraging that we are at last using more intelligence to feed ourselves. Organized medicine is now recognizing the worth of nutritional and preventive methods of treatment — and even of 'complementary medicine'!

It is also very encouraging that, whereas a short time ago the individual refused to accept responsibility for his own health, today there is an insatiable demand for any kind of self-help health care that offers an alternative to the orthodox answer of drugs.

As a result, alternative medicine and self-help groups are springing up, such as the Wessex Healthy Living Foundation in Bournemouth — the first in the country where attendant doctors and therapists give their services free in order to reduce the cost of consultation and treatment for the patient; the Healthy Life Association in Ipswich which now has branches in Felixstowe and Harwich; the Cancer Advice Clinic in Brighton; and the Cancer Help Centre in Bristol, opened by a very interested Prince Charles in July 1983. In his opening speech His Royal Highness urged that unorthodox medical treatment should not be dismissed as 'hocus-pocus'.

The authors of this book therefore feel that at no time could 'a new look at the Hay System' be more appropriate. People are ready to listen to the rationality and truthfulness of its precepts as never before. And the rewards are great; few people who have conscientiously investigated the principles of correct food combinations and correctly applied them to their eating habits have failed to experience tangible results in a very short time. Dr Hay reported: 'Thousands have found the mode of life so superior to anything they have ever before experienced that few ever return to less scientific modes of living, but continue to make the eating of their daily foods a scientific study because they have found that this pays better dividends than anything they have before encountered.' He also reported that while enthusiastic about their state of health they nearly all admit being deeply impressed with their *freedom from fear of disease in the future*.

Dr Hay has special words of advice for all enthusiastic devotees of the Hay System that are worth repeating. He told them *not to say too much about it*; not to make the mistake in their enthusiasm of trying to convert friends or relatives; not to force 'saving knowledge' on the unwilling; to help when help is desired; and by their own good health, efficiency and youthful appearance to be the most effective advocates — far better than reams of arguments — for the truths of right eating.

The distinguished actor, Sir John Mills, CBE, is just such an advocate. When asked in a press interview some years ago how he looked 'so astoundingly good at seventy,' and why he had 'hardly put on a pound in thirty years,' he replied: 'I've followed the same diet for thirty years — the main rule is do not mix protein with starch.'

Another famous film star, Evelyn Laye, was also a devotee of the Hay System. In the *Sunday Graphic* of 23 August 1936, she told how she adopted this way of eating when working in Hollywood and thoroughly upset because of a prolonged period of eating the wrong kinds of food: 'In a day I felt an improvement. In two weeks I was on tip-toe with health and vitality and felt more wide awake and energetic. I am certain that the reason for so many minor ailments in later life, such as indigestion, nerves, and those fits of what our kinder friends term "temperament" can be laid at the door of wrong eating in earlier days.'

It is an interesting fact of high importance and significance that it is not the body but the brain that shows the first evidence of improving nutrition, and often does so 'in a day' as Evelyn Laye and many others have experienced. As Dr Hay pointed out, clear thinking and right thinking both depend far more on the right foods eaten in the right way than people dream of in the average philosophy. There is no doubt whatsoever that our present-day nutrient-deficient, processed and junk foods are responsible to a considerable degree for the great increase in many of Society's present ills: serious personality problems in young children; ugly 'temperament' in home, office and factory; depression-caused suicides; broken marriages; juvenile delinquency; mental illness; appalling muggings and ever more violent crime. The psychological effects of food are powerful and far-reaching and this is only now beginning to be understood.

It is therefore encouraging that the disastrous, psychological effects of our late twentieth-century diet are at last being thoroughly investigated. In *The Times* of 1 August 1983, Barbara Griggs reported, in an article headlined *Sugar's Bitter Harvest*, that in the past two or three years researchers in America have been looking for possible links between the many polluting and nutrient-destroying factors in our diet and the growth of violent crime. *These researchers have found that sugar is 'the arch-criminal of the piece.'* Its over-consumption can result in the condition known as hypoglycaemia, or low blood sugar, 'in which messages from the brain controlling mood, motivation and learning are perpetually disrupted.' 'The result,' she wrote, 'may be a sudden burst of temper, aggression, changes of mood, confusion, fatigue and irritability . . . caffeine, alcohol, smoking and exposure to allergens can all trigger this unbalancing of the body chemistry, but *nothing triggers it faster, or more predictably, than sugar.*'

Barbara Griggs pointed out — as I too have pointed out many times elsewhere — that the rise in sugar consumption has exactly paralleled the rise in violent crime. Significantly, a study in America in 1980 'showed that a large percentage of juvenile delinquents tested were found to be eating more than 400 pounds of sugar a year in various forms.' Predictably, Professor A.J. Vlitos, Director General of the World Sugar Research Organization, the lobby for the world sugar industry, dismissed any evidence against sugar as 'flimsy'!

The new interest in the sugar/crime hypothesis is evident in the fact that 'Nutrition and Mental Health' was the theme of the 1983 McCarrison Conference held at St Hugh's College, Oxford on 23-25 September, with the approval of the World Health Organization. One of the speakers, Dr Michael Colgan, cited studies showing that criminal behaviour can be caused by bad food and prevented and treated by good food. Another speaker, Dr Alexander Schauss, clinical criminologist and author of *Diet, Crime and Delinquency* (Parker House, 1981), urged that both commercial concerns and government should work with academicians in order to assess the true impact of diet on deviancy, behaviour and learning.

In *Man the Unknown*, Nobel Prize-winner Dr Alexis Carrel made two profound observations which are highly relevant to the present argument: 'There is no doubt that consciousness is affected by the quantity and quality of the food . . . The possession of natural health would enormously increase the happiness of man.' In the light of these observations the Hay System offers an important and wholly beneficial dimension not only for avoiding degenerative disease, but for successful, healthy and happy living.

4.

BUTTER — NOT MARGARINE

The total fat consumption of Western man today is far too high for health and the medical establishment is advising the public to reduce it. *The Hay System, properly carried out, automatically reduces the consumption of all fats*. Unfortunately, the public is being brainwashed by propaganda into believing that butter and other animal fats are conducive to heart disease and should be replaced by margarine and vegetable oils. The authors of this book do not believe that animal fat is the villain of human nutrition and have used dairy products throughout the recipe sections in Parts Three and Four; they believe that natural, unprocessed, fresh foods are the basis of health, and so cannot on any account advocate the completely unnatural, highly processed spreads and oils now being manufactured and sold for human consumption.

Just how grossly processed are these spreads and oils is described by Ross Hume Hall, Professor of Biochemistry, McMaster University, Canada, in his thoroughly researched and well documented book, *Food for Nought*.[1]

Briefly: the seeds — soya bean, cottonseed, rapeseed, and corn — have first of all to be shatted to release the oil. This is done mechanically or with chemical solvents. The latter is the preferred method because it releases more of the oil from the seeds. The chemical solvent is boiled off, but traces up to 100 parts per million remain in the oil. These have to be reduced to the 'permitted' level — about ten parts per million. Depending on the source, however, the oil may contain undesirable 'free fatty acids'. These have to be removed by treating the oil at 140°-160° F with a solution of lye (caustic soda!). When the soap that forms settles out, the oil is skimmed off. It is then bleached — then subjected to a deodorizing process for about twelve hours! Finally, it is treated with an antioxidant to retard oxidation — *rancidity*. The antioxidant is usually 'butylated hydroxyanisole'. (Antioxidants, which are used to prevent rancidity in many products, are made from petroleum and are considered by some authorities as possible cancer-inducers.)

In order to harden the oil into spreads it has to be subjected to a process known as hydrogenation. For this the oil has to be mixed 'with a fresh or previously used nickel catalyst and subjected to hydrogen gas in a pressure reactor.' This process, however, leaves up to fifty parts per million nickel catalyst in the product. These used to be left in the oil, but now a 'scavenging' process is required to remove the nickel as traces of this catalyst have been found to make the product more susceptible to oxidation. 'The refining process,' warns Ross Hume Hall, 'leaves the oil almost completely devitalized . . . For example, lecithin has been expurged; this natural substance is associated with fatty materials in their natural state. It is an emulsifying agent, and aids in the digestion of fat.'

Professor Hall warns that physicians are promoting the eating of commercially processed vegetable fat in lieu of butter and other animal fats, 'knowing nothing of what they recommend.'

Quite apart from the massive *chemical* treatment, the *high heat treatment* of oils and spreads is alone sufficient to condemn them as nutritionally inadequate foods. According to Dr Norman Walker, 'if the fats have been treated in excess of 120° F, they will fail to be adequately treated by the pancreatic digestive juices and will not be available for use by the liver . . . thus their constructive nutritional value is destroyed.'[2] Yet many people have complete faith in the 'constructive nutritional value' of margarine. They little know that many margarines are made of just those highly saturated fats they think to avoid, and that the added colouring may be both carcinogenic and allergenic causing hyperactivity in their children.

The 'Fat Hypothesis'

The concept of eating these highly processed spreads and oils as a prevention against heart disease became a widely embraced medical dogma in the early 1970s, but it imposed much needless worry and very real anxiety upon millions of people. It is evolutionarily, epidemiologically, biologically and historically unwarrantable — *especially historically*. In the early part of this century, when margarine was little used, coronary disease was almost unknown. It was still a rare disease in the 1920s. From then onwards there was a steep rise in its incidence. According to one of Scotland's foremost heart specialists, in 1924 there were no cases of coronary heart disease (CHD) in his wards; but by 1954 there were over 300.[3] CHD is now occurring in increasingly younger men.

According to the Medical Correspondent of the *Sunday Telegraph* of 20 March 1983, fatal heart attacks among businessmen in their late twenties and early thirties have been reported by the worldwide medical emergency service Europ Assistance. This service — which guarantees on-the-spot medical aid for British subscribers travelling abroad — 'handled 115 fatal heart cases in the twenty-eight to thirty-six age group last year, compared with eighty-two cases in 1981, and seventy-three in 1980.'

The anti-animal-fat, low cholesterol diet which enjoyed such a cult in the 1970s is now largely in disrepute. Recent studies have so failed to vindicate the 'fat hypothesis' that there is now a remarkable medical turnaround, especially in the U.S.A.

An impressive example of this change in medical thinking is revealed by Dr George V. Mann in the *New England Journal of Medicine*, 22 September 1977. He asserts that 'A generation of research on the diet-heart question has ended in disarray . . . Foundations, scientists and the media, both lay and scientific, have promoted low fat, low cholesterol, polyunsaturated diets, and yet the epidemic continues unabated, cholesteremia in the population is unchanged, and *clinicians are unconvinced of efficacy.*'

Another example of this turnaround is contained in a report in May 1980 by the National Academy of Science and the National Research Council of America (considered the supreme court of science) which states that prevention of coronary heart disease cannot be achieved by means of dietetic or drug reduction of cholesterol, and its recommendation is that these measures should now be abandoned![4] Diet-conscious Americans received a big shock. And the members of the Food and Nutrition Board which produced the report were severely castigated as if they were heretics — *for recommendations which were so out of line with federal government agencies.*

Yet another example has been provided by one of the original promoters of the low-fat, low-cholesterol hypothesis, Professor Jens Dedichen of Oslo. He has frankly admitted that the Norwegian policy to reduce fat intake for the past twenty-five years — for which he was personally responsible — has produced *no fall in coronary mortality but rather a steady increase,* and this despite a five-fold increase in Norway in soybean oil consumption. He also admitted greatly regretting the anxiety created in the population by his policy and that during these twenty-five years it had become increasingly clear 'that we are on the wrong track.'[5] For this admission, needless to say, he was severely censured by his fellow scientists.

Professor Dedichen's findings have been confirmed

by numerous studies which failed to produce convincing evidence of the 'fat hypothesis', and which, moreover, claimed that although high blood cholesterol is *associated with* coronary heart disease it does not *cause* CHD.

The latest study, and by far the largest and most important one of all, was made in the U.S.A. It was called the MR FIT study (Multiple Risk Factor Intervention Trial), cost seventy million pounds, lasted ten years, and involved two groups each of 6000 men. One group was told to stop smoking, reduce saturated fats, eat more polyunsaturates, and take a drug to reduce blood pressure. The other group, serving as the control, was given no specific advice. The result became available in 1982 and is of the highest significance: after seven years there was no difference in mortality from heart disease between the two groups. [6]

This result, and those of many similar studies, have convinced many medical men of the fallacy of the 'fat hypothesis'. But its zealots still continue to promote it even, in some cases, to the point of fanatical absurdity. In the U.S.A., for instance, Coca-Cola is 'now being recommended for young Americans in order to avoid those dangerous saturates in milk'! [7]

The Dangers of Low-Fat, Low-Cholesterol Diets
Clinical trials of these diets have not produced the good that was expected of them and have produced evidence of harm that was not expected of them. For instance:

● There have been reports from the U.S.A. of increased malignancy in people eating polyunsaturated fats (highly processed vegetable oils and spreads). [8]

● Five patients who had all enthusiastically followed a diet-heart régime, substituting polyunsaturated margarine for butter, and polyunsaturated oil for cooking, developed malignant melanomas (a form of cancer).[9]

● There have been a number of reports linking low-fat and low-cholesterol diets with gallstone formation.[10] According to Professor Borgström, an outstanding leader in fat biochemistry, 'a diet rich in polyunsaturated fats will increase the risk of gallstones.'[11]

● A sharp rise in deaths from heart disease was reported in America between 1909 and 1961, during which time there was also *a sharp rise* in the consumption of unsaturated fats and oils.[12]

● Recent findings have shown that too drastic a reduction of cholesterol 'may lead to adverse changes in ageing cells so that they may not withstand the assault of incipient non-heart ailments.' So wrote Dr Cedric Carne in the *Sunday Express* of 13 February 1983, adding that 'it has recently been discovered that cholesterol may protect us from non-heart diseases'! He also wrote in the *Sunday Express* of 10 February 1974 that the belief that eating margarine and vegetable oils reduces cholesterol and prevents heart disease is '*the great medical myth of our time.*'

Animal fat — in moderation — is not the villain of modern-day diet after all!

Cholesterol is Vital for Health
Professor Ross Hume Hall has stated that 'cholesterol is a requirement of every living cell and we cannot live without it. It is the building block of sex hormones.'[1] Cholesterol also helps to make bile acids for digestion.[13]

It is not *the amount* of cholesterol, however, that is important but *the disturbed equilibrium between cholesterol and lecithin*. The latter emulsifies fats — helps to prepare them for absorption. There is no harm in foodstuffs containing natural cholesterol as, for instance, eggs, whose yolks though very rich in cholesterol are also high in lecithin and, at the same time, rich in vitamins and minerals. Such is the present obsession in America with cholesterol that there is now a dietary cult which demands that the nutrient-rich egg yolk is thrown in the garbage can and the white, only, retained for eating. As the egg white is a protein of doubtful use for the body, this is surely a case of throwing out the baby with the bathwater! It is significant that diet studies have revealed that 'adding two eggs daily to or withdrawing them from the diet had no effect at all on serum cholesterol levels.'[14]

Cholesterol and Vitamin C

In *Science* (16 February 1973) a highly important study by Dr Emil Ginter of the Institute of Human Nutrition in Bratislava, Czechoslovakia, has revealed that vitamin C is an important link in the conversion of cholesterol into valuable bile acids, and that a *lack* of vitamin C can cause high serum cholesterol and promote the onset of atherosclerosis. According to Dr Ginter's study, increasing vitamin C means more bile acids and this means that cholesterol remains in solution and does not precipitate out as gallstones or arterial 'plaque'.

In *The Lancet* (11 December 1971) research by pathologist Constance Spittle of Pindersfield Hospital, Wakefield, Yorkshire, also revealed the importance of vitamin C to cholesterol and bile acids. Her experiments to test the relation of vitamin C intake to serum cholesterol levels produced highly interesting results. In healthy people under twenty-five years of age, mean cholesterol levels dropped during a period of vitamin C therapy, but in atherosclerosis patients vitamin C therapy led to a pronounced rise in cholesterol. Dr Spittle believed this was due to 'the mobilization of arterial cholesterol' — in other words the life-threatening, hardened cholesterol in arterial plaque was loosened and washed out by the action of vitamin C. According to these results vitamin C could therefore be a specific therapy not only for *preventing* athero-sclerosis but also for effectively treating it even where the disease is advanced.

Judging from the findings of both Dr Ginter and Dr Spittle, if there is plenty of vitamin C in the diet — *such as in the high vegetable and fruit régime recommended in this book* — the fats required by the body can be eaten and metabolized so that they cause neither gallstones, nor atherosclerosis, nor any other trouble.

Fat is Vital for Health

The late Adelle Davis, an outstanding American nutritionist, has described how important fat is to health, especially for the proper functioning of the gall-bladder.

In *Let's Eat Right to Keep Fit*, she wrote: 'A certain amount of fat is necessary to stimulate the production of bile and the fat-digesting enzyme, lipase. Only when fat enters the intestine does the gall-bladder empty itself vigorously. Without fat (i.e. *natural* fat) too little bile is formed and the gall-bladder holds its reserve bile. This faulty emptying may be a factor contributing to the formation of gallstones.'[15]

Fat is also vital for the absorption of the fat soluble vitamins, A, D, E and K. Without the presence of fat and bile these vitamins cannot be carried across the intestinal wall into the blood.

It must be repeated: naturally occurring fat is not the villain in the modern-day diet.

Refined Sugar is the Villain

Since the early days of this century, nutritionally-minded doctors, dentists and scientists have given many authoritative warnings that refined sugar is damaging our health. But these warnings fell on deaf ears until the 1970s, when the research and writings of Surgeon Captain T.L. Cleave (R.N. ret'd) and his co-workers and converts produced evidence *as never before* that refined sugar and other refined carbohydrates such as white bread and flour were creating an epidemic of diseases which were wrecking the human body.

It is Dr Cleave's revolutionary concept that most diseases that are plaguing modern man are just different manifestations of one master disease which he terms 'the saccharine disease' (saccharine being pronounced like the river Rhine, and having nothing to do with saccharin, the chemical sweetener). This concept has been hailed as one of the most important medical discoveries of this century, both here and abroad, and has been responsible for an astonishing change in medical thinking regarding the importance in our diet of fibre-rich food such as wholewheat bread and bran.

The term 'saccharine disease' refers to all those conditions which Cleave advances as due to the taking of sugar, either primarily as such, or secondarily via the digestion of starch in white flour and other refined carbohydrates. These conditions constitute a formidable list of sugar-linked diseases, *including coronary disease*. Significantly, the steep rise in CHD since the early part of this century has been concurrent with an enormous increase in sugar consumption. But there has not been a similar enormous increase in fat consumption, although there has been an appreciable increase in this also. This increase, it should be pointed out, has not been in butter and other animal fats but in the highly processed margarines and cooking oils arbitrarily ingested in so many present-day foods: potato crisps, the ubiquitous chips with everything, including the 'chip butties' served at school meals, instant foods, pastries, cakes, ice-creams (of which increasing *millions* of gallons are now consumed yearly), biscuits etc.

The recent slight decrease in CHD deaths reported in the early 1980s has therefore been attributed to this increased consumption of processed fats. Since the 1960s, however, there has been *a marked decrease* in the consumption of sugar. There has also been *a marked increase* in the consumption of fibre-high wholewheat bread and bran. Thus *total* refined carbohydrate has decreased in the last twenty years. *This is the factor most likely to be responsible for the recent reduction in CHD deaths, and not that of increased margarine and plant oil consumption.* This conclusion is in perfect agreement with Dr Cleave's concepts.

In his book, *The Saccharine Disease,* [16] he puts forward irrefutable arguments and evidence which make a nonsense of the 'fat hypothesis'. He reveals the fallacy of treating coronary disease as an isolated disease and stresses that it is one of a group of interrelated diseases, often occurring with others — diabetes and obesity in particular — in the same patient. He is completely confident that 'the key to causation of coronary thrombosis lies in the causation of diabetes (and also of obesity).' He is equally confident that the 'absolutely dominant cause' of both diabetes and obesity lies in the over-consumption of refined carbohydrates, sugar especially, where the loss of fibre deceives the appetite and sense of satiety, and also causes an abnormally swift and massive absorption.

It is this clinical association with diabetes and obesity which so precisely indicts sugar, not fat, as the cause of heart disease. That fat is not the cause is confirmed by the freedom from coronary disease which has been carefully observed, and documented, in certain East African tribes, the Masai[17] and the Samburu, [18] despite diets containing enormous quantities of animal fat by our standards.

Fibre is the Crux of the Argument
As the fibre content of the diet goes up, so the blood level of

cholesterol goes down. This has been confirmed by experiments in animals and humans.[1] Fibre-rich foods therefore constitute an important protective factor against coronary disease.[19]

Regrettably, the obsession with cholesterol levels has blinded the 'fat' protagonists to the importance of a nutritionally adequate, high-fibre, wholefood diet. The whole focus of the 'fat hypothesis' has merely been on preventing coronary disease by means of *fat modifications*.

More regrettably, this obsession has delayed the recognition that such a nutritionally adequate diet not only offers a simple do-it-yourself means of preventing coronary disease and its clinically associated diseases, but also of preventing the many other manifestations of 'the saccharine disease'.

Dr Walter W. Yellowlees, Past President of the nutritionally-oriented McCarrison Society, scathingly summed up the complete absurdity of these 'fat modifications' when he wrote:

> Obession with cholesterol levels has led to some extraordinary dietary cults. These would have us substitute margarine for butter, restrict our egg consumption to three a week, and make the taking of cream a sin. (Whoever heard of anything so absurd as strawberries and skimmed milk.)[20]

There is, therefore, no need to refrain from using dairy products in the recipes set out in Parts Three and Four (unless for economy reasons or on doctor's orders), provided the refined carbohydrates are eschewed and the diet contains enough fibre-rich, and fresh, 'whole' foods.

1. Hall, Ross Hume *Food for Nought* (Harper & Row, New York, 1974)
2. Walker, N.W., *Natural Weight Control* (O'Sullivan Woodside & Company, Phoenix, Arizona, 1981)

3. Yellowlees, W.W., 'A General Practitioner's View' (Butter Information Council Seminar, January 1977)
4. McMichael, J., 'Dietary prevention of ischaemic heart disease', Correspondence, *British Medical Journal* (16 August 1980), p.517
5. Dedichen, J., *T. Norske Laegeforen* (1976) 16. 915
6. *Journal of the American Medical Association*, Vol 248, No. 12, (24 September 1982)
7. *World Medicine* (27 June 1981), p.21
8. *Medical News Tribune* (18 December 1971)
9. *Medical Journal Australia* (18 May 1974), p.810
10. *New England Journal of Medicine*, 228 (1):46 (1973)
11. Borgström, B., *Sartryk ur Livsmedeteknik* (1976) 7, 301
12. Yellowlees, W.W., 'A General Practitioner's View' (Butter Information Council Seminar, January 1977)
13. Pritikin, N., *The Pritikin Program for Diet and Exercise* (Grosset & Dunlap Inc., 1980)
14. Brisson, Germain J., 'Diet lipids and heart disease — A review of nutritional evidence', *Diet and Heart Disease* (Report of the International Symposium, London 1982)
15. Davis, A., *Let's Eat Right to Keep Fit* (Harcourt Brace and Company, New York, 1954)
16. Cleave, T.L., *The Saccharine Disease* (John Wright & Sons Ltd, Bristol, 1974)
17. *British Medical Journal* (31 July 1971), 3, 262
18. Shafer, A.G. et al., *East African Medical Journal* (1969), 46, 282
19. Trowell, H.C., *American Journal of Clinical Nutrition* (1972), 25, 926
20. Yellowlees, W.W., 'James McKenzie Lecture 1978', *Journal of the Royal College of General Practitioners* (January 1979)

5.

THE PROOF OF THE PUDDING . . .

Since the publication of this book we have received many letters from grateful readers, and we thought it would be interesting to include extracts from some of these in this new edition of the book. They provide fresh evidence of the remarkable — and often speedy — benefits experienced by readers on adopting the Hay lifestyle.

Two years ago at the age of 61 life became quite miserable, and diverticular trouble was diagnosed, also osteoarthritis in my knee . . . I tried a high fibre, low fat, sugar-free diet but still suffered with pain and the discomfort of an extended stomach. Then I tried to combine Dr Dong's arthritic diet with the high fibre diet, but this was still not the answer. In September a friend passed on some *Here's Health* magazines where I read of your Hay System. Suffice it to say that it is like a miracle. My weight is exactly correct for height now. A small but nasty warty mole on my left leg has completely disappeared, my stomach is normal and my arthritic knee improved unbelievably.

I am sure you'll be pleased to hear, as I am to tell you, that my health has improved a great deal since using your book. My arthritis has almost gone and I have much more energy.

Incidentally, it may interest you to know that I am an ex-Wimbledon player for G.B. for the last ten years in the Veteran classes (now over 70s). I am 75. Unable to play tennis for three months last summer I am now (Feb) playing quite well again!

Six months later this ex-Wimbledon player wrote: You may be pleased to hear that making your diet the foundation of my eating habits has helped me to regain perfect health, and although I am 75 have just entered for three tournaments in Spain in October.

For over twenty years I have been ill, overweight and desperately trying to 'diet'. I have followed endless diets, with limited success. I have been to an allergy clinic, which did help me with some of the problems I had been having with depression and irritable bowels, and I have been going to therapy sessions run by my G.P. to try to come to terms with the eating habits and chocolate addiction that were ruining my life. Now after following your advice I am delighted to find that my chocolate addiction has gone. Since I started to follow your ways, I have not eaten any at all, and I was previously trying to cut down on three *Mars* bars a day! I have not even wanted to eat chocolate, which is even more miraculous, and I was really hooked, and suffered the most trying withdrawal symptoms when I tried to give it up before. My headaches have gone, and I have been eating good amounts of food at each meal.

My husband and I (both in our late seventies and arthritic) enjoy an active and happy life, largely due, we are sure, to eating foods that do not fight, AND starting each day with cod liver oil and orange juice! We have recommended your book to many of our friends, with most beneficial results. One, who has suffered with a duodenal ulcer for many years, said it was 'like being reborn'. She now eats food denied to her in the past and now looks and feels a different woman.

An article in VOGUE magazine said that the Hay Diet would help a psoriasis sufferer. Imagine my delight when not only has my psoriasis almost cleared up, but I have lost approximately three stones in weight and feel much better and more alive than I have for years and years.

My sister, to whom I gave your book at Christmas, telephoned a few days ago. I asked her how she was and she said: 'Absolutely fine. I've just wheeled twelve barrow-loads of compost round the garden, and I couldn't wheel two before Christmas. I've lost 10 lbs and do not feel nearly so rheumaticky, I feel comfortable in bed and sleep so much better. I've tried all kinds of diet but never lost much weight and always felt hungry. In this way of eating I don't.' (By March, this 'sister' had lost over two stones in weight.)

The most remarkable case I've come across, and the nearest thing I shall see to a miracle, was a lady of seventy-two who was so badly crippled with arthritis that she was in a wheelchair and taken to hospital for treatment once a week by a specialist. Her hands were so deformed that they were permanently closed like boxing gloves . . . I suggested to her niece that she change her diet — not expecting her to do so for a minute. Six weeks later I casually asked her niece how her aunt was, fully expecting the worst because she was so ill that she couldn't move whilst lying in bed, and she was crying with pain when I last enquired. To my utter astonishment her niece replied: 'Oh, she's much better! She's actually written me a letter. Her pain has subsided greatly and she can move her hands enough to hold a pen,' and she showed me the letter.

I've met this arthritic lady twice since her recovery and she's walking perfectly normally. She also said that when she was better she was pushing a trolley around the supermarket one day when a young man suddenly stopped her and said: 'Excuse me, but is it Mrs Samson?' She turned and saw the young man who used to wheel her into the ambulance and take her to hospital for a weekly treatment. He looked as though he'd had a terrible shock and couldn't believe what he'd seen! (from a clinic for Alternative Medicine).

Equally convincing is the evidence from a busy general practitioner: 'You will be very pleased to hear that I am pursuing compatible eating both personally and in my practice, and with marvellous results on both fronts . . . In Jan/Feb I ate totally compatibly and lost my migraine of 20 years standing. Things happened and, while still eating compatibly much of the time, I let a very busy spell in the practice break my discipline, the diet lapsed, and my migraine returned. Six or seven weeks ago I took compatible eating fully on board again. I have now been migraine free for six weeks (the longest I can remember) and my hay fever cleared dramatically mid-season (right at the very worst time). The resolution of migraine and hay fever was most impressive.'

As I was desperate to find a remedy for indigestion (which was waking me up almost every night in the small hours) I decided to try — though without much hope of success — the Don't Mix Foods That Fight Diet. And now I have to confess — the results have been remarkable! Within two weeks I had lost six pounds in weight (which had been creeping on me into middle-aged spread!) without feeling the least bit hungry. The rheumaticky pains in my hands have improved, and neither my husband nor I have had a cold despite our office being full of them all winter long. I am so very grateful for being enlightened into sounder health and digestion.

I had suffered from indigestion for approximately 12 years and an ulcer or suspected ulcer had been diagnosed. In January of this year I was sent to hospital for a gastroscopy and was found to have a duodenal ulcer. I was placed on medication consisting of Zantac and

Gaviscon which relieved the symptoms at the time but if only one pill was missed I again suffered indigestion.

I was sent to a specialist who suggested an operation and took me off all medication for a month. Within two days the pain had returned with full intensity and at this stage I was only able to eat raw eggs, milk and cracker biscuits. Whilst on holiday I found *Food Combining for Health* and immediately started on the Hay System. Within the first week I was able to start eating more normally, and within two weeks could eat without suffering any indigestion whatsoever except on the starch meal, and I found the cause of this to be bread.

I returned to the hospital two weeks later, when I was asked if I wanted to be put on the medication, I declined the offer and also declined to undergo any form of surgery. It was suggested that I have a further gastroscopy which took place some three to four weeks later.

When I returned to the hospital for the results I was surprised to learn that they showed *no trace of the ulcer nor any signs of scar tissue.* Slowly over the last two to three months I have been able to eat perfectly naturally under the Hay System, even occasional meals of mixed starch and protein with no ill effect.

There is no doubt in my mind that I am already benefiting from the diet. It is years since I felt so well and happy. In fact now, at 60, I feel ten years younger than I did at 50 . . . My rescue is like a miracle, and I thank God daily for it when I happily tackle my household chores or go for long, long country walks. It's good to be alive and well and enjoying it all.

Three years ago I was seriously ill with aplastic anaemia, because my bone marrow was not making the red blood corpuscles I needed. I had no energy, could not walk far or do much, and some of my friends thought I was going to die.

Although my specialist gave me every care, she said *there was no cure in my case*, and I would need blood transfusions for the rest of my life. I had these in hospital every five and a half weeks, and the outlook seemed bleak.

But I would not accept the fact that I was incurable. For some time I had been searching for a healthy diet, particularly after reading *Your Daily Food*. So I went to a qualified naturopath, who put me on a diet which followed all your principles. Within three months, the time between transfusions gradually lengthened, until I lasted for 18 weeks. Then I had my twelfth and last transfusion. After 15 months from starting the diet, my bone marrow began to work again and my haemoglobin (red cell corpuscle count) gradually began to rise, and two years later is continuing to do so. I am so well that recently I was able to tour the Rockies in Canada, without fatigue. I am sure that the diet helped in my cure, and am eternally grateful.

When I received *Food Combining for Health*, I had already been diagnosed as suffering from an ulcer and treated with drugs. It was the busy season in our small shop and my complaint was causing severe disruptions and inconvenience . . . although apprehensive I was desperate to get away from the diet of 'little and often'. I am so glad I did — I have had no trouble since! There have been many completely unexpected additional benefits, the main ones being that within a few days I was relieved of a long standing and worsening condition of Colitis or irritable bowel (up to 5 or 6 times a day); indigestion cured immediately! I have lost 2 stones or so in weight over a period of time and feel a great deal better for it — all due to this book. I can see why people cannot believe it — it's so simple, so quick and effective that it sounds too miraculous to be true — yet all for the price of a couple of N.H.S. prescriptions. The real expense has been the acquisition of new clothes!

●   ●   ●

The experiences related in these letters, and in count-less others I have received, are convincing evidence of the inbuilt power of the body to heal, strengthen and restore. By removing many obstacles in the way of this healing power compatible eating releases the mar-vellous capacity of the body to renew itself and throw off disease.

PART TWO
THE HAY SYSTEM IN PRACTICE

by
Jean Joice

6.

HOW TO BEGIN

The joy of the Hay System is its flexibility; it is not a rigid diet to be endured but a delicious way of eating for health and well-being which can be enjoyed indefinitely.

Although this section of the book includes menus and recipes to help new converts to get started, it is hoped that readers will adapt their own favourite recipes and find new and imaginative ways of serving the wide range of delicious natural foods that are available season by season. There are now many books containing imaginative ideas for preparing the fruit and vegetables that are such an important part of the Hay System and some of these are listed in the Further Reading section at the end of the book.

The detailed chart of compatible foods on pages 139-141 will help you to assemble meals until this way of eating becomes second nature.

The rules of the Hay System, fully explained in Chapter Two, are very simple:

1. Starches and sugars should not be eaten with proteins and acid fruits at the same meal.
2. Vegetables, salads and fruits should form the major part of the diet.
3. Proteins, starches and fats should be eaten in small quantities.
4. Only whole grains and unprocessed starches should be used and all refined and processed foods should be eliminated from the diet. This particu-

larly applies to white flour and sugar and all foods
containing them, all highly processed fats such as
margarine and all highly-coloured and sweetened
foods and drinks such as orange squash.
5   An interval of four to four-and-a-half hours should
elapse between meals of different character.

The easiest way to put these rules into practice and to
achieve the ideal ratio of four to one between the
valuable alkali-forming foods (vegetables, salads and
fresh fruits) and acid-forming foods (meat, fish, eggs,
cheese and grains) is to arrange the day's meals so that
animal protein is eaten only once a day, cereal starches
are eaten only once a day, and the third meal contains
neither but consists only of fruit with milk or yogurt. It
is usually most convenient to take this essential
alkaline meal at breakfast, but, if a starch breakfast is
preferred, an alkaline meal consisting of salad, fruit
and yogurt could be taken either at midday or in the
evening. A comprehensive list of alkali-forming foods
is included at the end of the book to help you select
foods for this very important meal.

Another, perhaps unexpected, feature of the Hay
System is that although it excludes all highly processed
convenience foods, the time needed to prepare food is
usually far less than for the conventional cooked,
mixed meal. Meals are simpler and easier to prepare,
containing as they do a high proportion of raw fruits
and vegetables with their health-giving enzymes,
minerals and vitamins intact. Dr Hay emphasized that
simple meals are far better for health because they are
less taxing for the digestive system. The suggested
menus are, therefore, usually for two-course meals
consisting of one main dish with salad or freshly
cooked vegetables followed by fresh fruit in season.
The three-course meal consisting of starter, main
course and pudding should be regarded as an occasional treat for weekends, holidays or when enter-

taining. Those who give the system a fair trial will be surprised to find how satisfying and delicious this new way of eating can be, and how sugary 'treats', once relished, are no longer wanted.

On the following pages are listed the foods recommended for protein, carbohydrate and alkaline meals, and a 'black' list of foods to be avoided. Unfortunately this list is longer than when Dr Hay was writing because of the tremendous growth of food technology and the ever-increasing number of synthetic additives used in food processing. It is not only because of the many additives they contain that factory foods should be avoided but because they no longer retain their natural complement of fibre, vitamins and minerals *in their correct proportion to one another*. This is a most important factor which is often overlooked, for all natural wholefoods contain the micronutrients essential for their complete metabolism.

If the 'foods to avoid' list looks somewhat daunting, it is best to concentrate on the many delicious foods that *are* available in the recommended lists — many of these more readily available now than for many years thanks to an increasing awareness of the importance of the 'wholeness' principle in the growing and preparation of food.

THE FOODS TO EAT

Foods for a Protein Meal

Proteins
Meats of all kinds
Fish
Shellfish
Chicken
Game
Eggs
Cheese — the farmhouse
  variety, not processed
Nuts*
Mushrooms
Seeds*
Milk*** — fresh milk only,
  not homogenized or UHT
Yogurt

*Fats***
Butter
Cream
Egg yolks
Olive oil (cold pressed)
Sunflower seed oil (cold
  pressed)

Sugar substitutes
Concentrated apple juice
Diluted frozen orange juice
Honey in strict moderation
Maple syrup in strict
  moderation
Raisins and raisin juice*

*Vegetables**
All green vegetables
All root vegetables (but not
  potatoes)
Mushrooms
(Spinach and *cooked*
  tomatoes are best not

eaten more than once a
week because of their
high acid content)

Fruits
Apples
Apricots
Blueberries
Cherries
Grapefruit
Grapes
Guavas
Lemons
Lychees
Mangoes
Oranges — all kinds
Passion fruit
Peaches
Pears
Prunes (Santa Clara)
Raspberries
Strawberries

*Saladings**
Avocados
Beetroot (beet)
Cabbage
Carrots
Celery
Chicory
Cucumber
Fennel root
Legumes — sprouted
Mustard and cress
Lettuce
Parsley
Green peppers
Red peppers

Saladings (cont.)
Radishes
Seeds — sprouted
Tomatoes
Watercress

Salad dressings
French dressing
Cream dressing
Mayonnaise (homemade)
Use lemon juice or apple
  cider vinegar

*Note: Raisins, nuts, seeds, fats, saladings and vegetables combine with all meals.
**Fats: All fats are used in very small quantities and although cream is used in some recipes it is almost always used *instead* of another, possibly more concentrated, fat such as butter. If properly applied, the Hay System is a low-fat way of eating and automatically eliminates 'hidden fats'.
***Milk should be used sparingly by adults. It is intended by nature for young mammals! For adults it can be a great catarrh-former. It combines best with fruit and vegetables, and salads, but can be used in small quantities with starches and proteins, though not with meat.

Foods for a Starch Meal

Cereals and grains
Wholegrains: wheat; oats; barley; rice (brown, unpolished); rye; maize (corn); millet; buckwheat
Bread made from 100% wholemeal flour
Flour — 100% and 85% wholemeal

Sweet fruits
(All fresh fruits should be completely ripe)
Bananas
Custard apples
Dates
Figs (fresh or dried)
Grapes (only very sweet varieties)

Papayas (paw paw) (very ripe)
Pears (very sweet, and ripe varieties)
Raisins

Milk
Use in *moderate* amounts only

Eggs
Yolks only, but 'compromise' occasionally and use whole eggs

Fats
(As for a protein meal)
Butter
Cream

Fats (cont.)
Egg yolks
Olive oil (cold pressed)
Sunflower seed oil (cold
  pressed)

Vegetables
All green vegetables
All root vegetables
Potatoes (cooked in their
  skins and the skins eaten)
Pumpkins
Sweet potatoes
Mushrooms

Sugars
Honey
Molasses
Maple syrup (not synthetic)
Barbados sugar

(All sugars should be used
  in strict moderation.
  Avoid 'hidden' sugars
  such as those in
  commercial flavoured
  yogurt, bottled fruit
  drinks etc.)

Salad dressings
Sweet or sour cream
Olive oil (cold pressed)
Mashed uncooked tomato
  mixed with oil, paprika
  and seasoning

Unprocessed wheatgerm or
oatgerm and unprocessed
wheat or oat bran may be
taken daily

Foods for an Alkaline Meal
Acid fruits, milk or yogurt as listed for a protein meal.
All green and root vegetables; all salad vegetables; fats
as for a protein meal; seeds, such as sunflower seeds,
almonds, sprouted seeds and legumes.

A starch version of the alkaline meal can consist of
potatoes, cooked in their skins and the skins eaten,
served with butter and accompanied by a salad or
cooked green vegetables. For this meal any fruit to
finish should be selected from the list for starch meals.

Drinks
It is best not to drink at all with meals. The rule should
always be: drink only when thirsty. However, if it is
difficult to go without, the following suggestions may
help.

For a protein meal:
Weak tea or coffee (not instant) but no cereal coffee
substitutes. Ceylon tea such as Luaka which is low in

tannin or maté tea such as Yerbama are preferable to very strong teas. Herb teas are excellent. All teas should be taken without sugar.

Fruit juices made from fresh acid fruits preferably diluted with a little spring water. Apple juice with Perrier water makes a good thirst-quencher in hot weather and there are many excellent spring waters now available.

Do not drink milk with a meat meal. Milk should be regarded as a food not a drink and taken only in moderation.

For a starch meal:
Tea, coffee or herb teas as above and cereal coffee substitutes may be taken.

Fresh tomato juice and raw vegetable juices but not acid fruit juices. However, very sweet grape juice is permissible.

For an alkaline meal:
As for a protein meal. However, as milk combines best with fruit and vegetables it may be taken with a fruit breakfast.

Foods to Avoid
All refined carbohydrates. This means sugar in all forms, particularly white sugar and all food and drinks containing it.

It also means white flour and all foods made with it such as bread, cakes, biscuits, pastry and puddings; also white polished rice and other refined grains such as sago or tapioca.

Avoid aerated soft drinks, fruit-flavoured squashes and all bottled fruit drinks — even the so-called health drinks such as rosehip syrup or branded blackcurrant drinks, as these contain an appreciable amount of sugar. (One popular brand, undiluted, contains sixty per cent sugar.) Watch out in particular for 'hidden' sugars.

Read all food labels carefully, as sugar is contained in many foods where you might not expect to find it. Most muesli cereals, promoted as 'health foods', contain up to 26 per cent sugar. The 'high fibre' cereals are also high in sugar; most commercial ice cream contains over 20 per cent; tomato ketchup over 20 per cent and salad cream 18 per cent. Some sweet pickles contain over 30 per cent sugar; most fruit yogurts over 10 per cent and Cola drinks 10 per cent. Even the relatively innocent baked beans, containing no other additives, have a sugar content of 5 per cent, and many of the rusks on which babies cut their teeth contain up to 30 per cent sugar. Sugar is also contained in many toothpastes.

Most factory-produced and instant foods should be avoided because of the additives they contain. These are colourings, preservatives, flavour enhancers, emulsifiers and stabilizers added by food manufacturers to 'improve' appearance and flavour and to prolong shelf life. Although new synthetic additives undergo rigorous tests, no one really knows what the long-term effect on the human body may be, or what is the synergistic effect of an ever-increasing number. Many are under attack as the cause of hyperactivity in children. Highly-coloured foods are particularly dangerous in this respect.

The eight largest groups of additives are: flavours and flavour enhancers such as monosodium glutamate; thickeners and stabilizers; emulsifiers; food acids; colours; preservatives; anti-oxidants and sweeteners. The only safe rule is to read all food labels and avoid any product containing any of these additives. Unfortunately this is not so easy in the U.K. since many of these substances are now listed only by code. For example, the anti-oxidants BHA (butylated hydroxyanisole) and BHT (butylated hydroxytoluene) are now listed on food packets as E320 and E321 respectively. (In order to crack the code, read *E for Additives* by

Maurice Hanssen (Thorsons, 1984) which is a comprehensive guide to food additives and their code numbers). Since these substances were introduced in the early 1950s their safety has been in question. BHT in particular has been banned in many countries after tests indicated that it could lead to liver and kidney damage and increases in blood fat and cholesterol. It is still used in the U.K., though not in baby foods.

For a detailed and explicit account of the additives used in processed foods it is well worth reading *The Right Way to Eat* by Miriam Polunin (J.M. Dent, 1978); other foods to avoid because of additives are: dried fruit preserved with sulphur dioxide; and prepared meats, including bacon, containing sodium nitrate and sodium nitrite which in certain conditions can be cancer inducing.

Virtually all tinned foods should be avoided, battery eggs and chickens; pickles; legumes (unless sprouted); cranberries; rhubarb and plums (because of a high acid content). The use of salt should be reduced as far as possible and all heavily salted foods such as salted peanuts avoided altogether.

Fried foods should be omitted except for very occasional use. Instant coffee should never be used; tea or freshly-ground filtered coffee may be used in moderation.

Basic Essentials for the Hay System Larder
Fruit, vegetables and saladings. It makes good sense to buy only what you need for a short time ahead especially where fresh fruit and vegetables are concerned. If possible, buy organically grown vegetables or grow your own. Fresh foods start to deteriorate from the moment they are picked so buy the freshest you can find and store in the refrigerator, if there is room, or in a cool place until needed. All fruits and vegetables, especially from non-organic sources, should be thoroughly washed. In the case of apples and pears

etc., it is, alas, best to peel them.

Grains and stoneground wholewheat flours should also be kept in a cool place and used within three months or less. Whole grains and flours that contain the germ will not keep indefinitely and should always be used as soon as possible. The same thing applies to brown rice and wholemeal pasta such as macaroni and spaghetti and to seeds and nuts, particularly shelled nuts even when vacuum packed.

Fresh wheatgerm is a particularly valuable food supplement containing the vitamin B complex, vitamin E and EFA (essential fatty acids). Buy only from a supplier who has a fast turnover, and store in the refrigerator as it can go rancid very quickly. It can be sprinkled on cereals or used as a substitute for breadcrumbs in cooking.

Bran is another excellent addition to the diet though, if real wholewheat bread and plenty of vegetables are eaten, there should be enough fibre in the diet to solve any constipation problems without the need for additional bran. However, apart from supplying fibre, bran is also an excellent source of vitamin B_1, calcium and iron. It, too, should be stored in the refrigerator.

Steel cut oatmeal (medium) is useful for making a quick and delicious porridge and for making oatcakes. This is cheaper than packaged cereals and far more nutritious. Oatflakes can be used as a foundation for a homemade muesli.

Dried yeast for making bread. This keeps fairly well and is a good alternative to fresh yeast if this is difficult to obtain. The brand produced by the Distillers Company Ltd, known as D.C.L., is of consistently good quality.

Fats and oils. Use only fresh, unsalted or slightly salted butter and cold-pressed sunflower seed oil or good olive oil of first extraction.

The consumption of all fats should be decreased, and food should not be fried. The digestibility of a fat depends on its being heated as little as possible during processing. (All margarines are highly processed — see Chapter Four.) Fresh butter and vegetable oils contain the important EFA (essential fatty acids) factor, and the fat soluble vitamins A, D and E whose absorption depends on EFA. Summer butter and oils of first extraction have the highest content of vitamins A and E. Again, buy only what you need for immediate use and store in the refrigerator. Fresh butter can also be stored very successfully in the freezer.

Sea salt contains valuable trace elements but should only be used very sparingly. Most of us consume too much salt and should cut down on its use as much as possible. The use of dried or fresh herbs can help considerably to reduce the need for salt.

Honey. Provided it is organically produced and not blended with sugar, honey can be used occasionally as a sweetener.

Cider vinegar is the only vinegar which should be used for salad dressings. Malt vinegar should never be used.

Dried fruits can be very helpful as natural sweeteners, particularly raisins and dates, but do try to obtain fruit that has not been treated with chemicals. The sulphur dioxide used to preserve dried fruits destroys vitamin B_1 (thiamine) in the body and may interact adversely with other chemical additives. 'Sun-maid' raisins, which are sun dried and free of all additives, and date chips from organic suppliers make useful snack substitutes for children. If you cannot obtain organically grown sun-dried fruit be careful to blanch all dried fruit in boiling water and rinse again in cold water before using.

Natural whole brown rice is rich in vitamins B and E and

contains 300 to 400 per cent more of the B vitamins than polished white rice. Try to obtain organically grown brown rice. It has a far better flavour and is well worth the extra cost.

Yeast and vegetable extracts are excellent as spreads or for flavouring soups, casseroles or gravies. *Barmene, Natex* and *Vecon* are all very good.

Bread. Make every effort to bake your own bread using the quick Grant loaf method in the starch recipe section. Although the sales of 'brown' bread have risen in recent years, there is still much confusion about what is a genuine wholewheat loaf baked from 100% wholewheat flour. If you have a reliable baker you can check the ingredients but if you are not sure it is far better to be independent! Some of the chain bakeries are now producing wholemeal bread but these loaves also contain emulsifiers, permitted antioxidants and fat. Moreover the wholewheat flour from which the bread is made is not organically grown. Most good health food shops are now able to supply wholewheat flour from an organic source. Good bread, supplying all the naturally occurring vitamins, minerals and fibre contained in the whole wheat is absolutely fundamental to good health.

Meat, eggs and cheese. Happily there is a far greater demand now for meat that comes from animals reared naturally, without hormone implants or antibiotics in their feed. Obviously beef, lamb and chicken produced by traditional methods cost more but the meat tastes much better and, as you need less of it on the Hay System, the overall cost per week should not be any greater than with more frequent protein meals from the supermarket. It is worth making every effort to seek out organic producers of meat, chickens, free range eggs and farmhouse cheeses. *Thorsons Organic Consumer Guide*, (Thorsons, 1990), provides up to date information on where such good foods and fresh fruits and vegetables are to be found. Although fruit and some vegetables will not store, meat *can* be bought in bulk and frozen and it is well worth finding an organic producer of potatoes and other root vegetables in order to lay in a store for the winter if you cannot grow your own.

Potatoes are a 'convenience' food *par excellence*. They help to improve the diet by eliminating the use of too much cereal starch, and they contain more available calcium, phosphorus, iron and B vitamins than do milled cereals. In the Hay System they are promoted to a place of honour as a main dish accompanied by vegetables or salads; suggestions for potato meals are to be found in the starch recipe section. The most valuable part of the potato lies just below the skin. It has been reckoned that the average family throws away annually potato peelings equivalent in iron to 500 eggs, in protein to sixty steaks and in vitamin C to five glasses of orange juice. For this reason, try to obtain a supply of potatoes from an organic grower. They store well in a cool, dark place so you can buy enough at one purchase to last through the winter. Better still, if you can, grow your own.

The flavour of organically grown potatoes is far superior to commercially grown ones and there is no danger that the skins will have been treated with anti-sprouting chemicals. If you are not sure about the origin of the potatoes you buy, make sure that the skins are *very* thoroughly scrubbed before cooking.

Nuts are best bought in the shell and shelled just before use. In this way they will store well for some time. Once nuts have been shelled they should be used as soon as possible as exposure to light turns their fat rancid. They do, however, freeze well.

Nuts are a very concentrated food containing fat and protein. They are unadulterated foods which can replace animal protein. The protein in ¾ oz (23g) of nuts is equal to 1 oz (30g) of meat or fish. Most nuts contain unsaturated fat; the exceptions are coconuts and cashew nuts, whose fat is saturated. All nuts contain carbohydrate as well as fibre. They are best combined with vegetables, salads or fruits.

One of the most valuable nuts is the sweet almond which contains practically no starch. It has a fat content of fifty to fifty-five per cent and about twenty per cent protein. Almonds are rich in magnesium, iron and potassium but low in sodium. The almond is classed as an alkaline food.

Other valuable alkaline nuts are hazelnuts and brazils. The sweet chestnut is also an alkaline food but contains a much greater proportion of starch and little protein or fat. Chestnuts cannot therefore be used to replace meat protein, and should not be combined with protein foods or acid fruits.

Peanuts, which are really a legume (and therefore not recommended), cashews, pecans and walnuts are acid-forming and all contain valuable amounts of protein. Pecans are particularly valuable as they are very easily digested and therefore especially good for elderly people. Though expensive, only 1½ oz (40g) are required to replace an average serving of meat. All nuts are a good source of vitamins B and E and contain calcium, phosphorus and potassium. Be careful of commercial nut butters which are usually made from highly roasted nuts and heavily salted. They are usually extremely acid-forming, especially peanut butter.

Seeds such as sunflower, pumpkin and sesame seeds are excellent sources of protein, essential fatty acids (EFA), vitamins, minerals and trace elements. They are rich in magnesium and calcium. Pumpkin seeds are rich in B vitamins, phosphorus, iron and zinc. Sesame seeds are particular rich in calcium and vitamin E. Sunflower seeds are also rich in vitamin E, as well as the B complex, iron, magnesium and zinc. In her book *The Joy of Beauty* (Century Publishing, London, 1983) Leslie Kenton suggests grinding equal quantities of sunflower, sesame and pumpkin seeds in a blender and storing them in the refrigerator. Add a dessert-spoonful of the mixed seeds to breakfast dishes. All these seeds make excellent between-meal snacks too. Buy only what you need for immediate use as they quickly turn rancid when exposed to the air.

Raw foods are vital. Eat as much of your food raw as you possibly can. Aim for at least one salad a day composed of raw fruit, green leaves and roots and as far as possible eat all fruit in its raw state.

Only raw foods yield their full complement of vitamins, minerals and fibre. Heat immediately reduces and often destroys completely the vitamin C content of fruits and vegetables as well as other valuable elements. Most people have far too little vitamin C in their diet. The body needs a constant daily supply if it is to retain its youthfulness in old age.

Many studies have demonstrated the cleansing and curative effect of raw food on the human organism. In particular it has been found that cooking destroys valuable enzymes in the plant cells which help in the digestion of raw food, thus relieving the intestinal tract and ensuring better assimilation. For many years raw food diets have been used in the Bircher-Benner clinic in Zurich for the treatment of arthritis and other conditions, and fresh raw salads and sprouted seeds and grains are an essential part of the therapeutic diet recommended by the Cancer Help Centre in Bristol. A recently published book *Raw Energy* by Leslie and Susannah Kenton (Century Publishing, 1984), reviews much of the scientific evidence that demonstrates how problems such as fatigue, stress, hypertension, arthritis and premature ageing can be reduced by adopting a mainly raw food diet and gives much sound, practical advice on how to follow this type of régime.

Sprouted seeds, legumes and grains. Fresh sprouts are a marvellous way of increasing your intake of vitamins and minerals because germinating seeds and grains increases their nutritional value. The vitamin C content of wheat berries increases sixty per cent during sprouting. Sprouts are delicious in salads and are easy to grow in a sprouting tray or jar at any time of the year so they are especially valuable in winter. The best seeds to sprout are alfalfa, mung beans, aduki beans, lentils, fenugreek or wheat.

To sprout seeds take a heaped tablespoonful of your chosen seeds or beans and put into a clean 2 lb (1 kilo) jam jar. Cover with lukewarm (not hot) water and leave overnight. Next day cover the jar with a piece of muslin or cheesecloth and secure with a rubber band. Then drain off the water and replace with fresh tepid water, pouring off the excess. The seeds should be rinsed and drained twice a day. The sprouts will be ready to eat when they are between ½-2½ inches (1-6 cm) long, depending on which seed you have used. In *The Raw Food Way to Health* by Janet Hunt (Thorsons, 1978) there is an excellent chapter on sprouting seeds with details of how to grow and use a great many different kinds.

Fresh herbs. Try to grow some fresh herbs; if you have no garden they can be grown in pots on the window sill. Parsley in particular should always be used fresh and makes a valuable addition to salads, vegetable dishes and egg dishes. It is particularly high in vitamin C and iron.

The use of herbs in salads and cooking can help to improve flavour, stimulate appetite and decrease the need for salt in food preparation. Herbs that can easily be grown in a small space are:

● Basil — an annual which is delicious in all tomato dishes, tomato salads, with courgettes (zucchini)

and beans. Should be used fresh.
- Winter savory — makes a compact bush; the flavour of the leaves enhances all bean dishes.
- Tarragon — delicious in chicken dishes; good in salads and mixes well with other herbs.
- Rosemary, sage and thyme can all be used dried but are easy to grow in a small space.
- Chives are a very useful herb for those who don't like strong onion flavours.

Though not strictly speaking herbs, mustard and cress can easily be grown on the kitchen window sill and make a valuable addition to salads or sandwiches.

Corn salad or lamb's lettuce can give another welcome crop of green leaves in winter. It can be grown outside or in pots or boxes on a window sill. Joy Larkcom's helpful and practical book *Salads the Year Round* (Hamlyn Paperbacks, 1980) will help indoor and outdoor gardeners to increase their range of herbs and salad plants.

Blueprint for the Hay System Meal Plan
For most people the easiest way to follow the Hay System is to make one meal a day consist of alkaline foods only, one meal of protein with salads, vegetables and fruit and one meal of starch foods with salads, vegetables and a sweet fruit.

The basic meal plan looks something like this:

Breakfast (Alkaline):
Fresh fruit in season — best of all is a well flavoured apple; a pot of natural live yogurt, preferably home-made, with a tablespoonful of wheatgerm; a hot drink such as weak tea, herb tea, maté tea, dandelion coffee or real coffee (not instant). If coffee is chosen it should be made from finely ground coffee beans using the

filter method, which keeps back undesirable coffee oils and acids, and served with hot milk (half and half). Coffee should be used in strict moderation. Black coffee is not recommended. Tea and coffee should be made with bottled spring water rather than tap water and on no account use fluoridated water. In some areas a water filter such as the Mayrei, Brita or Waymaster Crystal may be helpful and reduce the cost of bottled water but they do not filter out fluoride or nitrates from the water supply.

Midday (Starch):
Potatoes cooked in their skins, butter, cooked vegetables or a salad; one of the sweet fruits or a dessert from the starch recipe section.

Alternatively this meal can consist quite simply of home baked wholewheat bread with butter and a green salad or just a 'salad' sandwich. If bran is taken it should be included with this meal. It can be mixed with wheatgerm, a few raisins and a little milk. If more convenient it can be taken with the fruit breakfast but this is not ideal.

Evening Meal (Protein):
This meal can include vegetable soup (made without stock), a moderate portion of meat, fish, chicken, shellfish, eggs or cheese; a salad of fresh raw vegetables; cooked green and/or root vegetables but not potatoes. This can be followed by fresh fruit from the 'acid' class such as apples, pears, oranges etc. Do not add sugar to these. Only one protein dish should be served and the helpings should be moderate. When no starches are eaten at this meal, less protein is required and more is digested.

The above meals are interchangeable. If a starch breakfast is preferred, the midday meal can be the alkaline meal. Dr Hay suggested that very active people should have their protein meal at midday and the starch meal

in the evening as the starchy meal entails more digestion than the protein type. This need not mean cooking
at midday; a simple protein meal could consist of a
green salad with farmhouse cheese followed by fresh
fruit.

For people who are very sedentary or who have
special problems to overcome it is recommended that
the number of alkaline meals should be increased and
the number of meals containing concentrated protein
or cereal starch should be decreased. The best way to
do this is to have *two* alkaline meals a day and have
protein or starch for the third meal on alternate days.
An alkaline meal based on potatoes can be very valuable in these circumstances to replace the cereal starch
meal.

Points to Remember
Lastly the following points are important to remember
when starting to put the Hay System into practice:

- Avoid eating between meals. If you feel you *must* eat
  something try sunflower seeds. As well as being
  very good to eat they are an extremely rich source of
  protein, minerals, amino acids, enzymes and vitamins A, B complex, D, E and F.

- If doing without sugar is difficult at first, use for
  sweetening a teaspoonful or so of 'honey syrup'
  made by dissolving one tablespoonful of honey in a
  quarter pint of boiled and cooled water. Store in a
  screw-top jar. On no account should artificial sweeteners be used; they can quickly destroy vitamin C
  and eventually may cause liver damage.

- Don't drink unless thirsty, and not immediately
  before or after meals. If desired, a cup of weak tea,
  herb or maté tea, with lemon or a small teaspoonful
  of honey, can be taken at mid-afternoon. Once

established on a correct meal pattern, tea-time cakes and biscuits will no longer be 'compulsive'.

● Eat as freely as possible fresh vegetables, salads and fruits.

● Never eat when tired or mentally upset.

● Treat alcohol with great respect; it should be used in strict moderation. Don't drink sweet wines, sweet sherry, liqueurs and sugary cocktails. A good dry wine, however, is compatible with a protein meal and helps digestion. Whisky and gin are 'neutral' but beer is classed as a 'refined carbohydrate' and should be avoided at (or near) a protein meal.

● Above all, don't forget that however important it is to eat the right foods, exercise and rest, fresh air and sunshine, deep breathing and *positive thinking* are all essential to health.

7.

MENU PLANNING AND SUGGESTIONS

The menus and recipes that follow, from the authors'
personal collections, are not intended to be comprehensive. No recipes for plain roasts or grills are
included as these may be found in any standard
cookbook. Nor will you find any recipes for cakes,
biscuits or fried foods — those items that contribute so
much fat, much of it 'hidden', to our modern diet. You
will find that our recipes use butter and cream but the
amounts are small and, because the use of meat and
milk is restricted, the consumption of saturated fats is
automatically reduced.

The recipes themselves contain only compatible
ingredients and all the recipes in each section are
compatible with each other so that a correctly combined main meal can be assembled from the protein *or*
the starch section. However, it is very important to plan
your meals for the day so that alkaline foods always
predominate.

In his book *Building Better Bodies*, Dr Hay listed foods
in the following order of importance:

Fruits
Leafy greens and raw salad foods
Root vegetables
Grains
Proteins

He maintained that we only need protein in very small
quantities and that all the elements for human health
can be supplied by fruits, greens, roots and milk. He

contended that meat, eggs and even cereal foods are not essential and in large quantities they can over-stimulate and overburden the metabolism. He also stressed that complex dishes should be avoided and that the best meals are composed of simple dishes of unprocessed foods and limited to two or three items. So, although it is possible to compile a three or four course dinner menu from the protein section, it is better to plan the main meal of the day round a *single* main dish of *either* protein *or* starch with a salad and fresh vegetables followed by just a piece of fresh acid or sweet fruit. The dessert recipes are intended only for occasional use.

The seasonal menu plans have been compiled to show how the Hay System works over a week or so of family meal planning and include suggestions for breakfasts, main meals without meat, very simple or fast meals that are easy to prepare when time is short or you are feeling tired, meals that use leftovers and meals for entertaining. If you are the only Hay dieter in the family you can still follow the system but supple-ment the meals of non-Hay people with items that you yourself do not have, such as potatoes with meat meals. When entertaining or eating out it is best to plan your menu round a protein main dish. People won't even notice, if there are several different vegetables, that you haven't helped yourself to bread or potatoes, and at home you can plan a compatible dessert. If cornered, as it were, when eating out, take Sir John Mills' advice and simply ignore the pudding or any other item that is not compatible with your main course. In the words of Surgeon Captain Cleave, author of *The Saccharine Disease*, 'if you don't want it, don't eat it.'

About kitchen equipment, make sure that your cooking pans are *not* made of aluminium, which can produce chronic aluminium poisoning. If possible use stainless steel — though expensive it lasts a lifetime — pyrex or corningware. Similarly, if using kitchen foil for roasting, use it only as an *outer* wrapping, after the food has been wrapped in buttered greaseproof paper, because of the danger of lead contamination.

Freezing

Because many of the recipes are low in fat or use raw or only lightly cooked vegetables, most of them are not suitable for freezing. Where a dish will freeze well this has been mentioned in the recipe.

Seasonal Menus

The following menus make use of each season's fruits and vegetables as far as possible since this still makes sense in terms of what our bodies need at different times of the year. The meal plan allows for one main meal per day and one light meal in addition to breakfast. The midday and evening meals are interchangeable and the main Sunday meal allows for entertaining friends.

A = Alkaline
P = Protein
S = Starch

SPRING MENUS FOR ONE WEEK

	Breakfast	Midday	Evening
Sunday	A Grapefruit sections	P Roast chicken with wheatgerm stuffing (page 186) Savoury mushrooms (page 194) Celeriac purée (page 192) Fruit and raspberry dessert (page 197)	S Mixed vegetable soup (page 215) Oatcakes (page 251) and butter
Monday	A Orange sections and yogurt	P Packed meal of cold chicken slices between lettuce leaves Leftover mixed vegetable soup in thermos Fruit of choice	S Potatoes Dauphinois à la Hay (page 234) Green salad Date chips or soaked, dried figs
Tuesday	A Spiced apple with raisins (page 200) and yogurt	S Salad sandwiches Banana and sunflower seeds	P Celery, apple and raisin salad with slices of farmhouse cheddar cheese

Wednesday	**A** Soaked dried apricots and yogurt	**P** Cottage cheese with tossed green salad Pineapple yogurt (page 207)	**S** Rice Pilaff (page 230) Mustard and cress Banana cream (page 242)
Thursday	**A** Spiced apple with raisins (page 200) and yogurt	**S** Mushrooms on toast Mustard and cress Dates	**P** Grilled plaice Parsley butter Steamed broccoli spears
Friday	**A** Sliced banana with wheatgerm and yogurt	**S** Pecan and pasta salad (page 220) Oatcakes (page 251) and butter	**P** Leek salad (page 156) Vegetables with Scotch collops (page 176) Apricot mousse (page 202)
Saturday	**A** Bircher muesli (page 132)	**P** Stuffed eggs (page 181) Coleslaw (page 155) Fresh fruit of choice	**S** Jacket potatoes with mushroom filling (page 236) Green salad Frozen bananas (page 245)

SUMMER MENUS FOR ONE WEEK

	Breakfast	Midday	Evening
Sunday	A Fresh raspberries Yogurt	P Tomato and Parsley cup (page 149) Chicken with lemon (page 174) Courgettes de luxe (page 190) Green salad Sliced nectarines in a glass (page 203)	S Creamed mushrooms on wholewheat toast Date ice cream (page 243)
Monday	A Blackcurrants with honey and yogurt	S Aubergine pâté (page 224) on toast (or in sandwiches) Nuts and raisins	P Courgette and tarragon soup (page 148) Cold chicken Lettuce and green salad Sliced fresh apricots
Tuesday	A Sliced fresh apricots with yogurt	P Green salad with sliced cheddar cheese	S Wholewheat pasta shells with parsley sauce (page 228) Frozen bananas (page 245)

Wednesday	A Fresh sliced peach with yogurt	S Tabbouleh (page 219) Watercress Fresh grapes	P Creamed cauliflower cheese (page 183) Tomato salad with fresh basil (page 158) Cherries
Thursday	A Raspberries and redcurrants with yogurt	P Mixed vegetable salad with curd cheese Cherries	S New potatoes baked with butter and parsley Garden peas and sliced courgettes Baked honey custard
Friday	A Sliced fresh apricots with yogurt	S Sandwiches of salad greens and savoury butter (page 253) Dates (packed meal)	P Grilled lemon sole and parsley butter Grilled tomatoes Green salad Raspberry and redcurrant compôte with cream
Saturday	A Fresh strawberries with yogurt	S Broad bean and savory salad (page 221) Wholewheat rolls with cream cheese	P Spanish omelette (page 178) Green salad Fresh peaches

AUTUMN MENUS FOR ONE WEEK

	Breakfast	Midday	Evening
Sunday	A Sliced apples and raisins with yogurt	P Roast topside of beef Cauliflower and brussels sprouts Carrot and white beetroot salad (page 161) Baked stuffed apples with cream (page 201)	S Baked potatoes with crispy skins (page 238) Green salad Dates and nuts
Monday	S Raw oatflakes with sliced bananas and milk	A Coleslaw (page 155) Pears and yogurt	P Cold roast beef Top favourite all-seasons salad (page 152) Sliced oranges
Tuesday	A Sliced apple and yogurt sprinkled with wheatgerm	P Waldorf salad (page 155) Stewed apricots	S Potato cakes (page 239) Ratatouille (page 189) (enough for two meals) Fresh figs

Wednesday	**A** Sliced pear and yogurt	**S** Salad sandwiches with savoury butter (page 253) Bananas (packed meal)	**P** Grilled lamb chops Ratatouille (page 189) Green salad Russet apples and walnuts
Thursday	**A** Sliced apple and yogurt sprinkled with wheatgerm	**P** Cream of celery soup Cottage cheese and orange salad	**S** Vegetable casserole (page 232) Dates and nuts
Friday	**A** Sliced grapefruit and yogurt sprinkled with grated hazelnuts	**S** Cress and cream cheese sandwiches Very sweet grapes (packed meal)	**P** Grilled Cornish mackerel Green salad Frozen strawberry mousse (page 199)
Saturday	**A** Sliced pear and yogurt	**P** Avocado salad à la Guacamole (page 154) with cheddar cheese Apple and raisin pudding (page 201) with cream	**S** Spaghetti with pesto (page 227) Ginger bananas (page 243)

WINTER MENUS FOR ONE WEEK

	Breakfast	Midday	Evening
Sunday	A Fresh grapefruit and orange sections	P Chicory, walnut and lamb's lettuce salad (page 160) Roast lamb Brussels sprouts Celeriac purée (page 192) Fresh pineapple slices	S Potato soup (page 214) Oatcakes (page 251) with butter
Monday	A Shredded raw apple with wheatgerm and yogurt	S Baked jacket potatoes with butter Mustard and cress Sliced tomato	P Leek and cauliflower soup (page 145) Cold roast lamb Red cabbage, apple and hazelnut salad (page 159) Sliced oranges
Tuesday	S Oatmeal porridge (page 252) with top milk	A Mixed vegetable soup (page 215) Carrot and raisin salad (page 222)	P Creamed cauliflower cheese (page 183) Green salad with sprouted seeds Fresh fruit

	A		
Wednesday	Soaked dried apricots with wheatgerm and yogurt	**P** Celeriac soup (page 213) Cheddar cheese Apples (packed meal)	**S** Rice with leeks and cashew nuts (page 229) Mustard and cress Sliced banana with sesame seeds
Thursday	Sliced apple and raisins with yogurt	**P** Mixed green salad Individual herb omelettes Oranges	**S** Vegetable casserole (page 232) Buttered cabbage (page 193) Fresh grapes
Friday	Soaked dried figs with wheatgerm and yogurt	**S** Banana and date salad (page 223) Wholewheat bread and butter	**P** Oven Baked sole (page 172) Savoury mushrooms (page 194) Green salad Apricot and apple fool (page 201)
Saturday	Bircher muesli (page 132)	**P** Celery, apple and raisin salad (page 157) with Almond balls (page 184)	**S** Hazelnut roast (page 233) Bean sprout and lettuce salad

Main Meals Without Meat
The alkaline and starch meals present no problems for the vegetarian but the following suggestions for protein main meals without meat may be helpful.

1. Spanish Omelette (page 178)
    Green salad with French dressing
    Fresh Fruit

2. Avocado salad à la Guacamole (page 154) served with thin slices of Cheddar cheese
    Fresh pears (peeled and sliced) served with Apricot sauce (page 209) and sprinkled with toasted sesame seeds

3. Stuffed eggs (page 181)
    Leek salad (page 156)
    Baked stuffed apples (page 201) with cream

4. Thick mixed vegetable soup (page 215) topped with grated cheese
    Fresh fruit

5. Almond balls (page 184)
    Coleslaw (page 155)
    Pineapple yogurt (page 207) or fresh fruit

6. Creamed cauliflower cheese (page 183)
    Top favourite all-seasons salad (page 152)
    Frozen strawberry mousse (page 199)

7. Waldorf salad (page 155)
    Hot apple and raisin pudding (page 201) with cream

8. Scrambled tofu on aubergine toasties (page 185)
    Fresh fruit

Breakfasts
Breakfast should always be a light meal. Dr Hay regarded it as superfluous but, if this seems too drastic,

limit breakfast to a light meal of fresh fruit only or fresh fruit and milk or yogurt. This provides the alkaline meal which is so important. If however you prefer a starch breakfast, this can be based on fresh whole cereals and sweet fruits.

Suggestions for both types of meal are listed below:

Alkaline Breakfasts:
- Any fresh acid fruit in season (see compatible food chart) with milk or yogurt.
- Fresh grapefruit or orange juice.
- Grated apple with one tablespoonful of wheatgerm and yogurt.
- Sliced fresh fruit and yogurt topped with sunflower seeds.
- Soaked dried apricots with yogurt and one table-spoonful of wheatgerm.

Note: Bran and wheatgerm may be added to the alkaline breakfast breakfast if desired. They are regarded as neutral since their starch content is negligible.

Muesli
Muesli is now a very popular breakfast dish but unfortunately the commercial 'muesli' mix bears no relationship at all to the original raw fruit porridge devised by Dr Max Bircher-Benner for his patients. Modern mueslis are essentially starchy cereal mixes whereas in Dr Bircher-Benner's muesli, grated raw apple or other acid fruit predominated and only a *level tablespoonful* of fresh rolled oats or medium oatmeal was permitted. Because the cereal content is so small and also because it is raw, freshly-made muesli, prepared according to Dr Bircher-Benner's recipe, may be regarded as an alkaline meal, and the recipe is given below. However, if you prefer a *mixed cereal* dish this is *not* muesli and should be regarded as a starch meal to be combined with one of the sweet fruits.

Dr Bircher-Benner's Muesli
1 *level* tablespoon rolled oats or medium oatmeal
3 tablespoonsful water
1 tablespoonful lemon juice
3 tablespoonsful raw milk if obtainable or natural
   yogurt
7oz (200g) apple (2 medium apples)
1 tablespoonful grated almonds or hazelnuts

1. Soak the oats or oatmeal with the water overnight.
2. In the morning, add the lemon juice and grate the
   well-scrubbed apples into the mixture and sprinkle
   the grated nuts on top.
3. Serve at once.

Starch Breakfasts
● A helping of mixed raw cereals (such as *Brown's* or
  Prewett's Muesli base) topped with one tablespoon-
  ful wheat bran and two teaspoonsful raisins. Soak in
  three tablespoonsful of water overnight. Serve with
  milk.
● Wholewheat toast with butter and a little honey.
● Poached or scrambled egg yolks on wholewheat
  toast.
● Millet flakes with sliced bananas and milk.
● Home-made oatmeal porridge.
● Soaked dried figs with mixed whole cereals and
  milk.
● Raw oatflakes, soaked overnight, served with sliced
  banana and milk.

Note: All cereal dishes may have bran and/or wheatgerm added to them if desired.

Practical Suggestions for Special Problems
Special health problems have been discussed in Part
One, but those who are tackling the following condi-
tions may find these suggestions helpful:

Allergies
When adopting the Hay System, allergy sufferers may find it easier *at first* to continue omitting the foods to which they are intolerant.

As allergy sufferers become established on compatible eating, however, they will find very quickly that they are no longer intolerant to any good, unprocessed food, or to natural substances in the environment.

Arthritis
The diet of arthritis sufferers should have a comprehensive vitamin and mineral supplementation. There are, however, three outstanding needs:

Vitamin C — it stimulates the production of hydrocortisone, the chief hormone where arthritis is concerned, and is also related to the nutrition of the joints.
Pantothenic acid (B5) — like vitamin C, it is vital to the normal production of cortisone and other adrenal hormones. According to Dr Roger Williams — the scientist who was the first to identify, isolate and synthesize pantothenic acid — it may be important in *preventing* arthritis.
Cod liver oil — This not only supplies vitamins A and D, and iodine, but also furnishes the means necessary for fixing lime (calcium) in the body. A tablespoon should be taken daily, on an empty stomach, an hour before a meal or four hours afterwards. It should also be emulsified for greater effectiveness according to the following instructions:

Place one tablespoon of pure, unflavoured cod liver oil in a small glass jar (such as a vitamin jar). Add two tablespoonsful of freshly squeezed orange juice (frozen orange juice is not suitable) and shake for a few seconds. Swallow quickly. Surprisingly, the orange juice completely masks the unpleasant taste of the oil. Milk can be used instead of orange juice but does not mask the taste.

The cod liver oil should be taken daily till the pain subsides. Then every second day for the next three months. After that, take once a fortnight — indefinitely. Apart from its beneficial effect on arthritis, it is an excellent tonic for both health and beauty, and retards the ageing process.

Indigestion

This condition, as shown in Part One, Chapter Three, will subside rapidly by means of compatible meals. But it will subside even more rapidly if a tablespoon of wheatgerm is taken at each meal. Wheatgerm is an excellent source of the B vitamins which help digestion and are especially necessary for the digestion of starch foods. Although wheatgerm contains the principal part of the protein of grains, the amount of this protein is insignificant. Wheatgerm can therefore be taken with any meal.

Sleeplessness

People who suffer from this condition should endeavour to make the last meal of the day as simple as possible, consisting of one course, but in amply satisfying amount. A protein meal is preferable to a starchy one. Coffee and strong tea should be omitted from the diet. Coffee, if insisted upon, should be restricted to one cup per day, diluted with milk or cream, and taken in the early part of the day. B vitamins in the form of wheatgerm, brewer's yeast and calcium pantothenate should supplement the diet. Calcium and magnesium, in the form of dolomite, are also very helpful.

Overweight

To speed up the process of losing weight, a fruit and milk breakfast should be preferred. A mixture of freshly squeezed orange juice and milk makes a delicious and satisfying drink. This mixture is not indigestible as so many people erroneously believe; the orange juice actually enhances the digestion of the milk.

If you lead an active life the protein meal is best taken at midday as the starch meal requires more digestion than the protein meal. Only a very moderate helping of the protein dish should be taken but you can also have a vegetable soup, salad, root and/or green vegetables with fresh fruit to follow.

The starch meal is best based on whole grains or potatoes. Bread in any quantity, and indeed most cereal starches, are best avoided while you are trying to lose weight. A potato meal as described in the starch recipe section accompanied by a salad and/or green vegetables is the best kind of starch meal for the overweight.

If you lead a fairly sedentary life try to have *two* alkaline meals per day, i.e. breakfast as above and the midday or evening meal consisting of salad, vegetables and fruit. Meat should be limited to once or twice a week.

Burping
Food repeats if the combinations of the meal have been wrong, and if it has had a habit of repeating for a long time, burping may persist for some time after the combinations have been corrected.

Gas
This indicates that too much acid-forming food has been eaten daily for too long a time. When the body chemistry is even approximately normal, natural foods seldom if ever disagree with one. This condition will quickly disappear when meals are correctly combined.

The Alkaline Meal
Because the alkaline foods should predominate in the diet they are an essential part of *every* meal in the form of the salads, vegetables and fruits that accompany

protein or starch dishes. However, the easiest time to fit
in a wholly alkaline meal is usually at breakfast and
suggestions for this are to be found in the breakfast
section (page 131).

Alkaline main meals can be composed of green or
root vegetables either steamed or cooked conservatively with a little water and served with a little butter
or cream, accompanied by any salad combination of
raw vegetables, sprouted seeds, saladings and/or fresh
acid fruit. Follow with fruit or sunflower seeds. A
starch version of the alkaline meal can consist of a
baked jacket potato with a little butter, a green salad
with a dressing appropriate to a starch meal and a
cooked green vegetable. This can be followed by one of
the sweet fruits listed for a starch meal. If, however, a
potato meal is taken as the alkaline meal no other starch
meal should be taken that day.

The list of alkali-forming foods at the end of the book
will help in assembling wholly alkaline main meals,
and the following list of easily prepared salads shows
what tremendous variety can be introduced into the
concept of the alkaline meal.

Twenty Fruit and Vegetable Salads for Alkaline Meals
- Chopped apple, chives and cabbage
- Grated carrot, apple and raisins
- Chopped apple and celery with cress
- Grated beetroot and onion with shredded cabbage
- Grated celeriac with sliced red and green peppers
- Sliced tomatoes with chopped fresh basil
- Sliced chicory (endive), sliced ripe pears and
  watercress
- Shredded white cabbage, apples and raisins
- Shredded red cabbage and orange sections
- Sprouted alfalfa (or other sprouted seeds), fresh
  parsley and chopped leek
- Chopped crisp radishes, sliced cucumber on
  shredded crisp lettuce

- Fresh peas cooked with mint served with shredded lettuce and some fresh, chopped tarragon
- Small courgettes (zucchini) grated and served with chopped chives and tarragon on shredded lettuce
- Cauliflower sprigs with cooked peas and sliced green peppers sprinkled with freshly chopped mint
- Diced fresh pineapple with tangerine sections and chopped mint
- Shredded white cabbage, diced pineapple and sliced green peppers
- Shredded tiny Brussels sprouts, diced celery and sunflower seeds
- Sliced cucumber, corn salad (lamb's lettuce) and chopped walnuts
- Shredded endive (chicory), grapefruit sections and chopped pecan nuts
- Diced beetroot (beet) chopped celery and chopped walnuts

With either basic French dressing: three parts oil to one part lemon juice. Shake in a glass jar with sea salt and freshly ground black pepper to taste and a little honey. For extra 'bite' add one teaspoonful Dijon mustard; *or simple cream or soured cream dressing*: single cream or soured cream seasoned with a little salt and paprika.

Miscellaneous Points
Animal fats. Two ounces (50g) of animal fat per day is believed to be the maximum allowance, and less than this would be advisable. Vegetable fats in the form of salad oils can be added to this allowance.

Melons are an excellent food, but are not easily digested with other foods. They are best taken on their own, when they make an excellent alkaline meal.

Peanut butter contains a great deal of starch along with a great deal of protein — as do all the legumes. It is therefore indigestible and acid-forming and is best used very infrequently. There are some delicious nut butters that can be used instead, such as *Sunwheel* Sesame Spread which contains just unhulled sesame seeds and sea salt, with no sugar or chemical additives.

Distilled water. Although this may be indicated in certain cases of stones or arthritis, it is not recommended for daily use. It is in what is termed a 'nascent state' when it is ready to take up any chemical with which it comes into contact, being wholly unsaturated. The best drinking water is a good spring water that is *not heavily mineralized*, such as *Malvern*, and *Highland Spring* from Scotland.

TABLE OF COMPATIBLE FOODS

Columns I and III are incompatible

can be combined   can be combined

I   II   III

For Protein meals	**Neutral Foods** can be combined with either Col. I or Col. III	**For Starch meals**
PROTEINS	NUTS	CEREALS
Meat of all kinds: Beef, lamb, pork, venison Poultry: Chicken, duck, goose, turkey Game: Pheasant, partridge, grouse, hare Fish of all kinds including shellfish Eggs Cheese Milk, including soya (combines best with fruit and should not be served at a meat meal) Yogurt, including soya	All except peanuts FATS Butter Cream Egg yolks Olive oil (virgin) Sunflower seed oil Sesame seed oil (cold pressed)	Wholegrain: Wheat, barley, maize (corn), oats, millet, rice (brown, unpolished), rye Bread 100% wholewheat Flour 100% or 85% Oatmeal — medium
FRUITS	VEGETABLES	SWEET FRUITS
Apples Apricots (fresh & dried) Blackberries Blueberries Cherries Currants (black, red or white if ripe) Gooseberries (if ripe) Grapefruit Grapes Guavas Kiwis Lemons Limes Loganberries Lychees Mangoes Melons (best eaten *alone* as a fruit meal)	All green and root vegetables except potatoes and Jerusalem artichokes Asparagus Aubergines (eggplants) Beans (all fresh green beans) Beetroot Broccoli Brussels sprouts Cabbage Calabrese Carrots Cauliflower Celery Celeriac Courgettes (zucchini) Kohlrabi Leeks	Bananas — ripe Custard apples Dates Figs (fresh & dried) Grapes — extra sweet Papaya (Paw paw) if *very* ripe Pears if *very* sweet and ripe Currants Raisins Sultanas VEGETABLES Jerusalem artichokes Potatoes Pumpkin Sweet potatoes

Columns I and III are incompatible

can be combined   can be combined

I	II	III
For Protein meals	**Neutral Foods** can be combined with either Col. I or Col. III	**For Starch meals**
FRUITS (cont) Nectarines Oranges Passion fruit Pears Pineapples Prunes (for occasional use) Raspberries Satsumas Strawberries Tangerines N.B. Cranberries, plums and rhubarb are *not* recommended	VEGETABLES (cont) Marrow (squash) Mushrooms Onions Parsnips Peas Spinach Swedes (rutabagas) Turnips	MILK & YOGURT only in moderation
SALAD DRESSINGS Fresh dressing made with oil and lemon juice or apple cider vinegar Cream dressing Mayonnaise (homemade)	SALADINGS Avocados Chicory (endive) Corn salad Cucumber Endive (chicory) Fennel Garlic Lettuce Mustard & cress Peppers, red and green Radishes Spring onions (scallions) Sprouted legumes Sprouted seeds Tomatoes (uncooked) Watercress HERBS & FLAVOURINGS Chives Mint Parsley Sage Tarragon Thyme	SALAD DRESSINGS Sweet or soured cream Olive oil or cold pressed seed oils Fresh tomato juice with oil and seasoning

Columns I and III are incompatible

can be combined   can be combined

I	II	III
For Protein meals	**Neutral Foods** can be combined with either Col. I or Col. III	**For Starch meals**
	HERBS & FLAVOURINGS (cont)	
	Grated lemon rind* Grated orange rind*	
	SEEDS AND SEED SPREADS	
	Sunflower Sesame Pumpkin	
	BRAN	
SUGAR SUBSTITUTE	Wheat or oat bran Wheatgerm or oatgerm	
Diluted frozen orange juice	SUGAR SUBSTITUTE	SUGARS
Concentrated apple juice	Raisins and raisin juice Honey Maple syrup	Barbados sugar Honey — in strict moderation
FOR VEGETARIANS (but not recommended)		
Legumes Lentils **Soya beans Kidney beans Chick peas (garbanzos) Butter (lima) beans Pinto beans **Tofu		
ALCOHOL	ALCOHOL	ALCOHOL
Dry red and white wines Dry cider	Whisky Gin	Ale Beer

*Use only organically grown fruit
**All soya products are processed; use sparingly

PART THREE
RECIPES FOR PROTEIN MEALS

8.

SOUPS AND STARTERS

LEEK AND CAULIFLOWER SOUP

Serves 4-6

Imperial (Metric)	*American*
2 leeks	2 leeks
1 oz (25g) butter	2 tablespoonsful butter
1 small cauliflower	1 small cauliflower
1 piece of mace	1 piece of mace
1¼ pints (700ml) water	3 cupsful water

1. Wash and chop the leeks.
2. Melt the butter in large pan and add the leeks.
3. Cook gently until the leeks are transparent.
4. Wash the cauliflower and divide into segments.
5. Add the cauliflower, mace and water to the pan and bring to the boil.
6. Reduce the heat and simmer for about 10 minutes until the cauliflower pieces are tender but not soggy.
7. Remove from the heat and liquidize until smooth.
8. Return to the pan and reheat. Season to taste.

TOMATO SOUP

Serves 4

Imperial (Metric)	*American*
1½ lb (700g) tomatoes	1½ pounds tomatoes
3 sticks of celery	3 celery stalks
1 onion	1 onion
1 medium carrot	1 medium carrot
1 oz (25g) butter	2 tablespoonsful butter
1½ pints (850ml) water	3¾ cupsful water
1 teaspoonful yeast extract	1 teaspoonful yeast extract
1 *bouquet garni* (sprigs of parsley, thyme, 1 bay leaf and 1 clove tied in a muslin bag)	1 *bouquet garni* (sprigs of parsley, thyme, 1 bay leaf and 1 clove tied in a muslin bag)
Sea salt and freshly ground black pepper	Sea salt and freshly ground black pepper
A little milk or single cream	A little milk or light cream

1. Skin the tomatoes by dipping them into boiling water for a minute, and cut into slices.
2. Wash the celery, onion and carrot and cut into slices.
3. Melt the butter in a thick-bottomed pan and add the vegetables.
4. Using a wooden spoon, stir and 'sweat' the vegetables for about 5 minutes.
5. Add the water, yeast extract, *bouquet garni* and the tomatoes. Bring to simmering point.
6. Cover pan and allow to simmer gently for 15-20 minutes.
7. Remove the *bouquet garni* and sieve the liquid or place in a liquidizer goblet and blend until smooth.
8. Return to pan and reheat.
9. Season to taste and add a little milk or cream.

MUSHROOM SOUP

Serves 4

Imperial (Metric)	*American*
1 oz (25g) butter	2 tablespoonsful butter
1 small onion, chopped	1 small onion, chopped
1 medium carrot	1 medium carrot
1 stick celery	1 celery stalk
8 oz (225g) large mushrooms	4 cupsful large mushrooms
1 heaped teaspoonful yeast extract	1 heaped teaspoonful yeast extract
1 pint (550ml) water	2½ cupsful water
Freshly grated nutmeg	Freshly grated nutmeg
Sea salt	Sea salt
Freshly ground black pepper	Freshly ground black pepper
4 tablespoonsful double cream	4 tablespoonsful heavy cream
1 tablespoonful dry sherry (optional)	1 tablespoonful dry sherry (optional)

1. Melt the butter in a large saucepan, add the chopped onion and cook very gently until golden brown.
2. Wash and slice the carrot, celery and mushrooms and add to the onion.
3. Add the yeast extract and water and bring to the boil.
4. Turn heat down to simmering point, cover pan and allow to simmer for approximately 15 minutes until the vegetables are just tender.
5. Pour mixture into a liquidizer and blend for 30 seconds until smooth; return to pan.
6. Reheat and add a miserly pinch of grated nutmeg (this gives a subtle flavour and also makes the mushroom flavour sing out).
7. Season to taste and just before serving add the cream.
8. For special occasions add the tablespoonful of dry sherry.

COURGETTE AND TARRAGON SOUP

Serves 4

Imperial (Metric)	*American*
1 lb (450g) courgettes	1 pound zucchini
1¼ pints (700ml) water	3 cupsful water
2-3 sprigs fresh tarragon *or* 1 teaspoonful dried tarragon	2-3 sprigs fresh tarragon *or* 1 teaspoonful dried tarragon
Sea salt	Sea salt
Freshly ground black pepper	Freshly ground black pepper
4 tablespoonsful soured cream	4 tablespoonsful soured cream

1. Wash and slice the courgettes (zucchini).
2. Put the water in a large pan and bring to the boil.
3. Put the courgettes (zucchini) and tarragon into the pan, bring back to boiling point and then reduce heat to a gentle simmer.
4. Simmer for about 5 minutes until the courgettes (zucchini) pieces are *just* tender but the outside skin should retain its bright green colour.
5. Remove from the heat and liquidize for 30 seconds until *almost* smooth but the green flecks of skin are still visible.
6. Return to the pan and reheat. Season to taste.
7. Pour into soup bowls and stir a tablespoonful of soured cream into each bowl. This soup is equally delicious hot or cold.

MINTED GRAPEFRUIT

Serves 4

Imperial (Metric)	*American*
2 large grapefruit	2 large grapefruit
Small handful of fresh mint leaves	Small handful of fresh mint leaves
2 level teaspoonsful honey	2 level teaspoonsful honey

1. Cut the grapefruit into halves and losen each segment with a grapefruit knife. Remove all pith from the centre of each half.
2. Wash, dry and chop the mint leaves finely.
3. Mix the mint with the honey and place a half teaspoonful in the centre of each half grapefruit.
4. Place the grapefruit halves in individual serving glasses and chill for 30 minutes.

TOMATO AND PARSLEY CUP

Serves 4

Imperial (Metric)	*American*
4 large *or* 8 small tomatoes	4 large *or* 8 small tomatoes
Fresh parsley	Fresh parsley
Sea salt	Sea salt
Freshly ground black pepper	Freshly ground black pepper
A little fresh basil	A little fresh basil

1. Skin and slice the tomatoes.
2. Wash, dry and chop the parsley.
3. Mix tomatoes and parsley (use a generous amount) and season with salt, pepper and a teaspoonful of freshly chopped basil. Use a pinch of dried basil if you have no fresh available.
4. Serve in individual cups.

MUSHROOMS IN SOURED CREAM

Serves 4

Imperial (Metric)	*American*
1 large tomato	1 large tomato
¼ pint (150ml) soured cream	⅔ cupful soured cream
1 teaspoonful lemon juice	1 teaspoonful lemon juice
1 tablespoonful finely chopped parsley	1 tablespoonful finely chopped parsley
8 oz (225g) small button mushrooms	4 cupsful small button mushrooms
Sea salt	Sea salt
Freshly milled black pepper	Freshly milled black pepper
Paprika	Paprika

1. Peel the tomato and chop finely, removing the seeds.
2. Stir tomato, lemon juice and chopped parsley into the cream.
3. Wash and dry the mushrooms and slice them.
4. Stir the mushrooms into the cream mixture and season to taste.
5. Spoon the mixture into individual glasses and dust with a very light sprinkling of paprika.
6. Chill for 30 minutes before serving.

COURGETTES VINAIGRETTE

Serves 4

Imperial (Metric)	*American*
8 small courgettes	8 small zucchini
1 teaspoonful sea salt	1 teaspoonful sea salt
1 large onion	1 large onion
6 tablespoonsful olive oil	6 tablespoonsful olive oil
3 tablespoonsful cider vinegar	3 tablespoonsful cider vinegar
½ teaspoonful Dijon mustard	½ teaspoonful Dijon mustard
½ teaspoonful clear honey	½ teaspoonful clear honey
Paprika	Paprika
1 tablespoonful chopped parsley	1 tablespoonful chopped parsley

1. Wash the courgettes (zucchini) and slice into rounds about ¼-inch (5mm) thick.
2. Put a little water and sea salt into a saucepan and bring to the boil.
3. Add the courgettes (zucchini) and allow to simmer gently for about 5 minutes until just tender but not soggy.
4. Drain well and allow to cool.
5. Slice the onion finely and arrange with the courgettes in individual bowls.
6. Mix the oil, vinegar, Dijon mustard and honey and pour over the courgettes (zucchini).
7. Sprinkle each bowl with a pinch of paprika and the chopped parsley.
8. Chill for 30 minutes before serving.

9.

SALADS, DRESSINGS AND SAUCES

TOP FAVOURITE ALL-SEASONS SALAD

Serves 4

Imperial (Metric)	*American*
4 tablespoonsful French dressing (page 162)	4 tablespoonsful French dressing (page 162)
1 lb (450g) firm white cabbage, shredded	4 cupsful shredded white cabbage
Other ingredients in quantities according to taste:	*Other ingredients in quantities according to taste:*
Red and/or green pepper	Red and/or green pepper
1-2 sticks of celery	1-2 stalks of celery
Freshly shelled walnuts, *or* cashew nuts *or* freshly skinned almonds	Fresh shelled English walnuts,*or* cashew nuts *or* freshly skinned almonds
3-4 extra-sweet dried apricots	3-4 extra-sweet dried apricots
1-2 apples	1-2 apples
Small piece of cooked beetroot	Small piece of cooked beet
Chives *or* grated onion	Chives *or* grated onion

1. Place the French dressing in a good-sized salad bowl.
2. Cut cabbage into thin shreds and intermix with the French dressing. (Cabbage is the best source of dietary fibre next to wheatbran.) This should be the base of the salad.
3. Skin and slice the pepper, chop the celery and add to the salad.

4. Add the nuts, and the dried apricots, both blanched and cut into thin strips.
5. Lastly cut up the apples, leaving the skin on if it is free from chemical sprays, dice the beetroot (beet) and chop the chives finely or grate the onion.
6. Mix all the ingredients well together, adding more dressing if necessary. The small piece of beetroot (beet) will give the salad a beautiful pink colour.

Note: The ingredients of this salad can be varied according to season but the base of the salad should always be the cabbage. The apple, too, is a vital ingredient — infinite variety can be achieved by adding one or more of the following:

Shredded Florence fennel root
Young garden peas
Sprouted seeds or mung beans
Chopped cucumber
Chopped mint leaves
Sliced radishes
Dried or fresh herbs
Raisins
Roughly chopped watercress
Fresh tarragon (superb!) snipped into small pieces
Parsley, snipped into small pieces
Carrot, cut into matchsticks, or coarsely grated for speed
Chopped celeriac
Quartered orange sections
Mustard and cress

The secret of a successful salad of this kind is to have as much variety in the texture of the ingredients and in the sizes of shredding as possible. It is important to be able to see the various ingredients and not to reduce the salad to an indistinguishable mush. Some shredding can be done with a sharp knife; other shredding is more effective on a stainless steel grater which has three different grades of shredding; some ingredients, such as chives and parsley, are best just snipped with kitchen cooking scissors.

AVOCADO SALAD À LA GUACAMOLE

Serves 4

Imperial (Metric)	*American*
2 large avocados	2 large avocados
Juice of a lemon	Juice of a lemon
2 tomatoes	2 tomatoes
2 sticks of celery	2 stalks of celery
½ red pepper, skinned	½ red pepper, skinned
½ onion *or* 1 shallot	½ onion *or* 1 shallot
1 clove garlic	1 clove garlic
1 dessertspoonful finely chopped parsley	2 teaspoonsful finely chopped parsley
2 tablespoonsful double cream	2 tablespoonsful heavy cream
Sea salt	Sea salt
Freshly ground black pepper	Freshly ground black pepper

1. Halve the avocados lengthwise. Remove the stones and scoop out the inner flesh leaving some adhering to the skin so that there is a thick firm shell remaining.
2. Rub a little of the lemon juice on the inner surface of the shells to prevent discolouration.
3. Cut the scooped-out flesh into dice, place in a bowl and stir in the rest of the lemon juice.
4. Skin, deseed and chop the tomatoes.
5. Chop the celery, red pepper and onion and add these ingredients and the tomatoes to the avocado in the bowl.
6. Add the garlic, squeezed through a press, parsley, cream and seasoning.
7. Combine the mixture well; it will thicken and make its own salad dressing.
8. Fill the shells and chill before serving.

Note: This salad makes a refreshing starter for 6 people if smaller helpings are served in individual pots.

Alternatively it can be served with thin slices of Cheddar cheese as a main course for 4, as a light midday or evening meal.

WALDORF SALAD

Serves 4-6

Imperial (Metric)	*American*
4 sticks of celery	4 stalks of celery
2 oz (50g) chopped walnuts	½ cupful chopped English walnuts
2 large dessert apples	2 large dessert apples
6 oz (175g) Cheddar cheese	1½ cupsful Cheddar cheese
¼ pint (150ml) Mayonnaise (page 165)	⅔ cupful Mayonnaise (page 165)
Sea salt and freshly ground black pepper to taste	Sea salt and freshly ground black pepper to taste

1. Chop the celery and walnuts.
2. Dice the apples and cheese.
3. Mix all together in a salad bowl and add mayonnaise.
4. Give a final mix, adding salt and pepper to taste.

COLESLAW

Serves 4-6

Imperial (Metric)	*American*
12 oz (350g) white cabbage	12 ounces white cabbage
8 oz (225g) carrots	8 ounces carrots
1 small onion	1 small onion
2 oz (50g) seedless raisins	⅓ cupful seedless raisins
½ pint (275ml) Mayonnaise (page 165)	1⅓ cupsful Mayonnaise (page 165)

1. Shred the cabbage, grate the carrots and chop the onion finely.
2. Combine all the ingredients in a salad bowl, add mayonnaise and toss well. For a lighter coleslaw, toss with French dressing (page 162).

LEEK SALAD

Serves 4

Imperial (Metric)	*American*
2 large leeks	2 large leeks
1 small green pepper	1 small green pepper
2 oz (50g) walnuts	1 cupful English walnuts
Sea salt	Sea salt
Freshly ground black pepper	Freshly ground black pepper
6 tablespoonsful French dressing (page 162)	6 tablespoonsful French dressing (page 162)

1. Trim and clean the leeks thoroughly and slice across finely.
2. Blanch the leeks in boiling water for 2 minutes, drain thoroughly and allow to cool.
3. Remove the core and seeds from the green pepper and slice finely.
4. Chop the walnuts.
5. Combine the leeks, green pepper and walnuts in a salad bowl and toss with dressing.

CELERY, APPLE AND RAISIN SALAD

Serves 4

Imperial (Metric)	*American*
1 head celery	1 head celery
2 red-skinned dessert apples	2 red-skinned dessert apples
2 oz (50g) raisins	⅓ cupful raisins
6 tablespoonsful Basic Soured Cream Dressing (page 164)	6 tablespoonsful Basic Soured Cream Dressing (page 164)

1. Wash the celery thoroughly and slice finely.
2. Scrub the apples *very* thoroughly and slice.
3. Combine all ingredients together and toss well with the dressing.

TOMATO SALAD WITH FRESH BASIL

Serves 4

The success of this salad depends on using the finest ingredients: if possible the large Continental tomatoes such as Marmande, *fresh* basil and the best quality olive oil.

Imperial (Metric)	*American*
1 lb large well-flavoured tomatoes	1 pound large well-flavoured tomatoes
1 clove garlic (optional)	1 clove garlic (optional)
2-3 spring onions	2-3 scallions
A good handful fresh basil leaves	A good handful fresh basil leaves
6 tablespoonsful French dressing made with cider vinegar and virgin olive oil (page 162)	6 tablespoonsful French dressing made with cider vinegar and virgin olive oil (page 162)

1. Peel and slice the tomatoes and arrange in a serving dish which has been rubbed with the cut clove of garlic.
2. Chop the spring onions (scallions) very finely and scatter over the tomatoes.
3. Chop the basil leaves finely and sprinkle over the tomatoes and onions.
4. Pour over the French dressing and leave for 10 minutes for the flavours to merge.

Note: Do not make this salad too far in advance or the tomatoes will become mushy.

RED CABBAGE, APPLE AND HAZELNUT SALAD

Serves 4

Imperial (Metric)	*American*
1 lb (450g) red cabbage	1 pound red cabbage
2 eating apples — Cox's or Russets are best	2 eating apples — Cox's or Russets are best
2 oz (50g) raisins	⅓ cupful raisins
4 tablespoonsful French dressing (page 162)	4 tablespoonsful French dressing (page 162)
2 oz (50g) hazelnuts, coarsely chopped	⅓ cupful coarsely chopped hazelnuts

1. Wash the cabbage and shred finely.
2. Core and chop the apples coarsely.
3. Combine cabbage, apple and raisins in a salad bowl, pour in the dressing and mix well.
4. Sprinkle chopped hazelnuts on the salad just before serving.

Note: This salad is best made between 1 and 2 hours before it is needed.

CHICORY, WALNUT AND LAMB'S LETTUCE SALAD

Serves 4

Imperial (Metric)	*American*
1 lb (450g) white chicory	1 pound white endive
3 heads of lamb's lettuce (corn salad)	3 heads of lamb's lettuce (corn salad)
2 oz (50g) fresh walnut kernels, coarsely chopped	½ cupful coarsely chopped, fresh English walnut kernels
4 tablespoonsful French dressing made with virgin olive oil (page 162)	4 tablespoonsful French dressing made with virgin olive oil (page 162)

1. Wash the chicory (endive) and lamb's lettuce and dry carefully.
2. Slice the chicory (endive) and place in a bowl with the walnuts.
3. Pour in the French dressing and turn the pieces in the dressing so that they are well coated.
4. Arrange the lamb's lettuce leaves on a serving dish and pile the chicory (endive) and walnuts in the centre. Pour over the remaining dressing and serve immediately.

Note: This is a salad for gardeners, as I have never seen lamb's lettuce, or corn salad as the seedsmen usually call it, in a greengrocer's. However, it is a marvellous winter standby, providing florets of small green leaves throughout the coldest winter. I always plant some in August to be sure of some green salading when nothing else is available.— J.J.

CARROT AND WHITE BEETROOT SALAD

Serves 4

Imperial (Metric)	*American*
8 oz (225g) grated raw white beetroot	1¾ cupsful grated raw white beet
8 oz (225g) grated carrot	1¾ cupsful grated carrot
3 tablespoonsful finely chopped parsley	3 tablespoonsful finely chopped parsley
¼ pint (150ml) Basic Soured Cream Dressing (page 164)	⅔ cupful Basic Soured Cream Dressing (page 164)
Sea salt	Sea salt
Freshly ground black pepper	Freshly ground black pepper

1. Mix the grated white beetroot (beet) and carrot together and add the parsley.
2. Pour over the basic sour cream dressing and check for seasoning. Add extra salt and pepper if needed.

Note: This is another salad for keen gardeners! Having hated dark red beetroot (beet) since childhood, mainly because in British 'salads' the juice usually clashed with the colour of the tomato, experiments with the white and golden beet varieties (now easily obtainable as seed) have proved very successful. The golden variety is particularly attractive and this salad could also be made with equal quantities of grated golden beetroot (beet) and apple, with a few raisins, using the basic sour cream dressing.

BASIC FRENCH DRESSING

Imperial (Metric)	*American*
1 level teaspoonful sea salt	1 level teaspoonful sea salt
½-1 crushed clove of garlic (optional)	½-1 crushed clove of garlic (optional)
1 teaspoonful Dijon mustard	1 teaspoonful Dijon mustard
2 tablespoonsful freshly squeezed lemon juice *or* cider vinegar	2 tablespoonsful freshly squeezed lemon juice *or* cider vinegar
Freshly milled black pepper	Freshly milled black pepper
6 tablespoonsful virgin olive oil *or* cold pressed sunflower seed oil	6 tablespoonsful virgin olive oil *or* cold pressed sunflower seed oil

1. Put all the ingredients into a screw-topped jar and shake vigorously.
2. This amount should be enough to dress two salads or more and can be stored in the refrigerator.
3. If a sweeter dressing is preferred, 1 teaspoonful of clear honey can be added to the basic dressing. If garlic is not liked, chopped chives can add an extra zest.

FAVOURITE 'SWEET-SOUR' DRESSING

Imperial (Metric)	*American*
1 small shallot *or* onion equivalent	1 small shallot *or* onion equivalent
1 small clove garlic, halved	1 small clove garlic, halved
1 teaspoonful cider vinegar	1 teaspoonful cider vinegar
1 teaspoonful lemon juice	1 teaspoonful lemon juice
1 rounded teaspoonful honey	1 rounded teaspoonful honey
1 teaspoonful dry mustard	1 teaspoonful dry mustard
1 slice of fresh red pepper, (about 1 oz/25g) cut up*	½ cupful fresh red pepper, cut up*
4 fl oz (125ml) sunflower seed oil or olive oil	½ cupful sunflower seed oil or olive oil
Pinch dried thyme or the equivalent fresh thyme	Pinch dried thyme or the equivalent fresh thyme
2-3 sprigs of parsley	2-3 sprigs of parsley
Pinch of sea salt	Pinch of sea salt

1. In a blender, or food processor fitted with the steel blade, place all the ingredients except the oil, and start the blending.
2. Then add the oil slowly through the feeder and blend till the mixture is smooth and of the consistency of thin mayonnaise.
3. Adjust seasoning if necessary and store in the refrigerator in a screw-topped glass jar till required.
4. It saves work to make double this quantity as it keeps well when refrigerated.

*This is an important ingredient.

BASIC SOURED CREAM DRESSING

Imperial (Metric)	*American*
¼ pint (150ml) soured cream	⅔ cupful soured cream
1 teaspoonful finely chopped onion *or* chives	1 teaspoonful finely chopped onion *or* chives
2 tablespoonsful lemon juice	2 tablespoonful lemon juice
1 teaspoonful English mustard powder	1 teaspoonful English mustard powder
1 teaspoonful honey	1 teaspoonful honey

1. Place all the ingredients in a liquidizer goblet and blend well together.

Variations:

Yogurt can be used instead of soured cream but is not so effective.

For dressing cabbage salads the addition of a half teaspoonful of yeast extract gives an extra zest.

MAYONNAISE

Imperial (Metric)	*American*
2 egg yolks at room temperature	2 egg yolks at room temperature
1 teaspoonful dry mustard	1 teaspoonful dry mustard
Pinch sea salt	Pinch sea salt
Freshly ground black pepper	Freshly ground black pepper
2 tablespoonsful cider vinegar	2 tablespoonsful cider vinegar
½ pint (250ml) cold pressed olive oil	1⅓ cupsful cold pressed olive oil
1 tablespoonful boiling water	1 tablespoonful boiling water

1. Put the egg yolks and seasoning into a blender.
2. Add the cider vinegar and blend ingredients together at the lowest speed.
3. Put the oil into a small jug, remove the centre cap of the blender and start to pour oil onto the egg mixture *very slowly* (almost drop by drop) keeping the motor at its lowest speed.
4. Continue to add oil very slowly until the mixture begins to thicken.
5. When the mixture has thickened, add the rest of the oil in a steady stream until it has all been taken up.
6. Lastly add the boiling water and switch the blender off.

EGGLESS MAYONNAISE*

Imperial (Metric)	*American*
8 fl oz (225ml) whipping cream	1 cupful whipping cream
1 teaspoonful clear honey	1 teaspoonful clear honey
¼ teaspoonful paprika	¼ teaspoonful paprika
½ teaspoonful sea salt	½ teaspoonful sea salt
8 fl oz (225ml) sunflower oil	1 cupful sunflower oil
2 teaspoonsful lemon juice	2 teaspoonsful lemon juice

1. Whip the cream until soft and fold in the honey, paprika and salt.
2. Using an electric whisk at slow speed, gradually add sunflower seed oil.
3. When the mixture begins to thicken add the lemon juice.

*With acknowledgement to *Tempting and Nutritious Recipes* (Natural Food Associates, U.S.A.)

PAPRIKA DRESSING

Imperial (Metric)

1 tablespoonful fresh
   lemon juice
3 tablespoonsful virgin
   olive oil *or* cold pressed
   sunflower seed oil
1 teaspoonful clear, mild
   honey (Acacia is best)
1 good pinch paprika
1 tiny pinch cayenne
   (optional)
1 level teaspoonful any
   herb mixture preferred
Sea salt
Freshly ground black
   pepper

American

1 tablespoonful fresh
   lemon juice
3 tablespoonsful virgin
   olive oil *or* cold pressed
   sunflower seed oil
1 teaspoonful clear, mild
   honey (Acacia is best)
1 good pinch paprika
1 tiny pinch cayenne
   (optional)
1 level teaspoonful any
   herb mixture preferred
Sea salt
Freshly ground black
   pepper

1. Place all the ingredients in a screw-top jar and screw lid on firmly.
2. Shake vigorously before using.

FRESH TOMATO SAUCE

Imperial (Metric)	American
1 medium onion	1 medium onion
1 lb (450g) fresh tomatoes, if possible the large Continental kind such as Marmande	1 pound fresh tomatoes, if possible the large kind such as Marmande
1 oz (25g) butter	2 tablespoonsful butter
½ pint (250ml) vegetable stock	1½ cupsful vegetable stock
1 crushed garlic clove	1 crushed garlic clove
1 tablespoonful tomato purée	1 tablespoonful tomato paste
1 small handful chopped fresh basil leaves	1 small handful chopped fresh basil leaves
Sea salt	Sea salt
Freshly ground black pepper	Freshly ground black pepper

1. Chop the onion; skin and chop the tomatoes.
2. Melt the butter in a large, thick-bottomed pan and cook the onion gently until transparent.
3. Add the remaining ingredients, bring to the boil.
4. Reduce heat and simmer for 20 minutes or so. Do not cover the pan.
5. Adjust seasoning if necessary.

Note: This is a good standby and can be stored in the refrigerator, or if you have a glut of home grown tomatoes it can be made up in larger quantities as it freezes well.

RED PEPPER SAUCE

Imperial (Metric)	*American*
8 oz (225g) red peppers, deseeded and roughly chopped	2 cupsful red peppers, deseeded and roughly chopped
2-3 large, unpeeled garlic cloves	2-3 large, unpeeled garlic cloves
6 tablespoonsful virgin olive oil *or* cold pressed sunflower seed oil	6 tablespoonsful virgin olive oil *or* cold pressed sunflower seed oil
1 dessertspoonful lemon juice	2 teaspoonsful lemon juice
Sea salt	Sea salt
Freshly ground black pepper	Freshly ground black pepper

1. Place the red peppers and garlic in a saucepan with just sufficient water to cover and simmer for about 10 minutes until the peppers are very tender.
2. Drain, skin the garlic cloves and blend the peppers and garlic in a liquidizer or food processor for a minute or so.
3. With the motor still running at low speed add the oil in drops, slowly, until the mixture has thickened, followed by the lemon juice.

Note: An excellent sauce for serving over skinned and sliced avocado pears. Slice these longways to make an attractive presentation. Can be used as a colourful starter for special occasions.

10.

MAIN DISHES

MACKEREL WITH SORREL OR GOOSEBERRY SAUCE

Buy small, absolutely fresh fish; clean them and score each side of the backbone three times with a sharp knife to allow the heat to reach the thickest part. Cook under a hot grill, allowing 4-7 minutes for each side. Place on a serving dish and keep warm while finishing the sauce.

Sorrel Sauce:

Serves 4

Imperial (Metric)	*American*
1 large handful sorrel leaves	1 large handful sorrel leaves
1 oz (25g) butter	2 tablespoonsful butter
¼ pint (150ml) single cream	⅔ cupful light cream
¼ pint (150ml) double cream	⅔ cupful heavy cream
Juice from cooking the fish	Juice from cooking the fish
Sea salt and freshly ground black pepper	Sea salt and freshly ground black pepper

1. Remove the stems from the sorrel and wash thoroughly.
2. Place the leaves and butter in a thick saucepan and let the leaves simmer gently in the melted butter until they are reduced to a purée (3-4 minutes).
3. In another saucepan heat the cream but do not let it boil. Stir in the sorrel purée and fish stock, made by adding a

little water to the pan in which the mackerel were grilled and bringing to the boil.

4. Season to taste and serve with the mackerel.

Gooseberry Sauce:

Serves 4

This is the classic sauce for mackerel.

1. Follow the above method substituting a purée of ripe dessert gooseberries for the sorrel. Use ½ lb (225g/2 cupsful) of gooseberries, washed and simmered with a little butter until they are soft enough to purée in a blender.

OVEN BAKED SOLE

Serves 2

Allow one medium sole for each person. Ask the fish-monger to skin the fish on both sides.

Imperial (Metric)	*American*
2 medium soles, skinned on both sides but left on the bone	2 medium soles, skinned on both sides but left on the bone
2 tablespoonsful butter	2 tablespoonsful butter
2 fl oz (60ml) dry white wine	¼ cupful dry white wine
2 fl oz (60ml) water *or* fish stock	¼ cupful water *or* fish stock
Juice of ½ lemon	Juice of ½ lemon

1. Preheat oven to 350°F/180°C (Gas Mark 4).
2. Season the fish and place in a well-buttered ovenproof dish.
3. Pour the wine, water/stock and lemon juice over the fish.
4. Bake for 15 minutes, basting from time to time.
5. Brown under a very hot grill (broiler) for 2 minutes.

POACHED FRESHWATER TROUT WITH CREAM AND PARSLEY SAUCE

Serves 4

Imperial (Metric)	*American*
4 trout	4 trout
4 pints (2.4 litres) water	10 cupsful water
6 tablespoonsful wine vinegar	6 tablespoonsful wine vinegar
2 bay leaves	2 bay leaves
10 black peppercorns	10 black peppercorns

1. Clean the trout as quickly as possible but don't rinse them.
2. In a large pan bring water and wine vinegar to boil and add bayleaves and peppercorns.
3. To serve hot, slip trout into boiling water and simmer for 5-10 minutes according to size until cooked. Serve with Cream and Parsley Sauce (below).
4. To serve cold, slip trout into boiling water, bring back to the boil, remove pan from heat and leave to cool.

Cream and Parsley Sauce:

Imperial (Metric)	*American*
2 oz (50g) unsalted butter	4 tablespoonsful unsalted butter
¼ pint (150ml) double cream	⅔ cupful heavy cream
Sea salt	Sea salt
Freshly ground black pepper	Freshly ground black pepper
1 tablespoonful finely chopped parsley	1 tablespoonful finely chopped parsley

1. Melt the butter in a thick-bottomed saucepan.
2. When it has melted, stir in the cream. Keep stirring over a low heat until the sauce bubbles.
3. Season with salt and pepper and stir in the parsley. Serve at once.

Note: A green salad to which has been added some shredded Florence fennel root goes very well with the cold trout.

CHICKEN WITH LEMON

Serves 4-6

Imperial (Metric)	*American*
1 good chicken (about 4 lb/2.3 kilos)	1 good chicken (about 4 pounds)
2 oz (50g) butter	4 tablespoonsful butter
1 lemon	1 lemon
1 onion stuck with a clove	1 onion stuck with a clove
A sprig of fresh tarragon — if not available use parsley	A sprig of fresh tarragon — if not available use parsley
Sea salt	Sea salt
Freshly ground black pepper	Freshly ground black pepper

1. Preheat oven to 425°F/220°C (Gas Mark 7).
2. Clean the chicken and put half the butter inside the bird with a piece of lemon peel, the onion, tarragon or parsley, a little sea salt and freshly ground black pepper.
3. Squeeze the lemon and coat the outside of the chicken with the lemon juice, a little salt and pepper.
4. Place the chicken on a large sheet of parchment baking paper* dotted with butter where the chicken is to be placed. Use the remaining butter to smear the breast and legs.
5. Pour over any remaining lemon juice and bring up the sides of the sheet of paper to enclose the chicken in a loose parcel. Enclose this in an outer sheet of foil. Do not seal too tightly.
6. Place in the oven and roast for approximately 1 hour.
7. Halfway through the cooking remove the bird from the oven and baste thoroughly. Open the top of the parcel for the last 10 minutes to allow the breast to brown nicely.
8. This chicken is equally delicious served hot with green vegetables or cold with a green salad.

*The use of parchment baking paper prevents any possible lead contamination from the foil.

COLD CHICKEN À LA HAY

Serves 4-6

Imperial (Metric)

American

1 young chicken	1 young chicken
1 *bouquet garni* (usually consists of 2-3 sprigs of parsley, 1 sprig thyme and 1 bayleaf tied in a piece of muslin for easy removal)	1 *bouquet garni* (usually consists of 2-3 sprigs of parsley, 1 sprig thyme and 1 bayleaf tied in a piece of muslin for easy removal)
2 egg yolks	2 egg yolks
½ pint (250ml) double cream	1⅓ cupsful heavy cream
Grated zest of a well-scrubbed lemon	Grated zest of a well-scrubbed lemon

1. Place the chicken in a large casserole with a *bouquet garni* and half fill with water. Poach carefully in oven at 350°F/ 180°C (Gas Mark 4) until done. (The time will depend on the size of the chicken.)
2. Remove from the oven and allow to cool.
3. Divide the chicken into several large pieces and arrange on serving dish.
4. Beat up egg yolks with cream and stir over low heat until slightly thickened, but do not allow to boil.
5. Pour over chicken and sprinkle with the grated lemon peel. The sauce will thicken as the dish cools. Serve with a mixed green salad.

Variation:

SIMPLE TARRAGON CHICKEN

A delicious variation of this recipe is a simple tarragon chicken. Instead of a bouquet garni, when poaching the chicken, use several sprigs of fresh tarragon and, after the final dish has cooled, sprinkle the chicken with finely chopped fresh tarragon instead of lemon.

VEGETABLES AND SCOTCH COLLOPS

Serves 3-4

Imperial (Metric)	*American*
1 dessertspoonful sunflower seed oil	2 teaspoonful sunflower seed oil
12 oz (350g) best lean steak, minced	12 ounces best lean ground steak
Seeds from 3-4 cardomom pods	Seeds from 3-4 cardomom pods
½ teaspoonful dried thyme	½ teaspoonful dried thyme
1 small piece well-scrubbed orange peel	1 small piece well-scrubbed orange peel
3 tablespoonsful water	3 tablespoonsful water
12 oz (350g) mixed vegetables roughly chopped, such as: 1 or 2 courgettes, 2 good-sized mushrooms, a large carrot, a piece of celeriac, 3-4 shallots *or* 1 onion, ¼ red pepper (more if liked)	2 cupsful mixed vegetables roughly chopped, such as: 1 or 2 zucchini, 2 good-sized mushrooms, a large carrot, a piece of celeriac, 3-4 shallots *or* 1 onion, ¼ red pepper (more if liked)
½ teaspoonful potato flour	½ teaspoonful potato flour
1 tablespoonful finely chopped parsley	1 tablespoonful finely chopped parsley
Sea salt and freshly ground black pepper	Sea salt and finely ground black pepper
For garnish:	*For garnish*:
4-6 tomatoes	4-6 tomatoes
1 teaspoonful chopped fresh basil (Use dried basil if fresh not available)	1 teaspoonful chopped fresh basil (Use dried basil if fresh not available)

1. Place the oil in a heavy-bottomed pan. When medium-hot add the minced steak, cardomom seeds, thyme and orange peel and stir with a wooden spoon until all the meat grains are separated.
2. Add the water and prepared vegetables and cover the pan. Simmer at a very low heat for 1½ hours. Add a little more water during cooking if necessary, but when cooked the water should be nearly evaporated.
3. Mix the potato flour with 1 teaspoonful water and stir into the mixture until it thickens slightly. Season and add chopped parsley.
4. Turn onto a serving dish garnished with grilled halved tomatoes which have been sprinkled with the chopped basil.

SPANISH OMELETTE

Serves 2

Imperial (Metric)	*American*
2 dessertspoonsful cold pressed olive oil *or* sunflower seed oil	4 teaspoonsful cold pressed olive oil *or* sunflower seed oil
8 oz (225g) prepared mixed vegetables such as sliced courgettes, a little chopped red and/or green pepper, chopped carrots, one or two sliced mushrooms	1¾ cupsful prepared mixed vegetables such as sliced zucchini, a little chopped red and/or green pepper, chopped carrots, one or two sliced mushrooms
1 tablespoonful finely chopped parsley	1 tablespoonful finely chopped parsley
Sea salt	Sea salt
Freshly ground black pepper	Freshly ground black pepper
3 whole eggs *and* 1 yolk	3 whole eggs *and* 1 yolk
1 oz (25g) grated mild Cheddar cheese	¼ cupful grated mild Cheddar cheese

1. Heat the oil in a heavy-bottomed pan.
2. Add the vegetables and stir for a few minutes over a medium heat until they start to sweat.
3. Turn the heat to very low and cook gently until tender but not mushy, stirring frequently.
4. At this stage stir in the chopped parsley and season with salt and pepper.
5. Lightly beat the eggs and egg yolk and add seasoning.
6. Preheat a 9-inch (23cm) diameter omelette pan, add 1 dessertspoonful oil and allow to become medium-hot (not smoking!).
7. Transfer the vegetable mixture to the omelette pan and spread evenly.
8. Pour the eggs onto the vegetable mixture and stir gently.
9. Continue to stir gently with a fork for half a minute or so until the omelette begins to set.

10. Top with the grated cheese and brown under a hot grill. Do not allow the omelette to become too firm in the centre.
11. Cut into two, loosen with the palette knife and slide onto a warmed serving plate.

Note: This is good with a green salad, watercress or home-grown mustard and cress.

Note: Cold stuffed omelettes make a delicious salad meal, summer or winter. The stuffings can be varied: grated cheese; herbs; creamed mushrooms; cooked peas.

INDIVIDUAL COLD SUMMER OMELETTES*

To make one omelette:

Imperial (Metric)	*American*
1 small tomato	1 small tomato
1 large egg	1 large egg
Sea salt	Sea salt
Black pepper	Black pepper
½ oz (15g) butter	1 tablespoonful butter
Chopped parsley	Chopped parsley

1. Skin, deseed, chop and season the tomato.
2. Break the egg into a bowl and stir firmly with two forks, adding a mild seasoning of sea salt and freshly ground black pepper.
3. Warm a 6-inch (10cm) omelette pan but don't make it too hot. Then turn the heat up to high.
4. Put the butter in the pan and when melted and just beginning to colour, pour in the egg.
5. Add the tomato mixture and using a fork make sure it is folded well into the omelette.
6. From this point Elizabeth David's instructions cannot be bettered:
   Tip the pan towards you and with a fork or spatula gather up a little of the mixture from the far side. Now tip the pan away from you so that the unset egg runs into the space you have made for it. When a little of the unset part remains on the surface the omelette is done. Fold it in three with your fork or palette knife, hold the pan at an angle and slip the omelette out onto the waiting dish.
7. Decorate with lots of chopped parsley.

*With D.G.'s grateful acknowledgement to Elizabeth David's *Summer Cooking* (Penguin Books).

STUFFED EGGS

Serves 4

Imperial (Metric)	*American*
4 eggs	4 eggs
Sea salt	Sea salt
Freshly ground black pepper	Freshly ground black pepper
1 teaspoonful yeast extract	1 teaspoonful yeast extract
Yogurt	Yogurt
Paprika	Paprika
Sprigs of parsley	Sprigs of parsley

1. Put eggs into a pan of cold water, bring to the boil and allow to boil for 10 minutes.
2. Pour off the water and allow the pan to stand under running cold water for a few minutes until the eggs are cold. (This prevents discolouration of the egg yolk.)
3. Shell the eggs and cut in halves lengthwise.
4. Remove the yolks and place them in a blender or food processor, adding the seasoning and yeast extract. Blend with sufficient yogurt to make a stiff but creamy mixture.
5. With a teaspoon neatly scoop out (and discard) some of the egg white in each half to enlarge the space for the filling.
6. Pile the egg yolk mixture into the scooped out shells and decorate with a sprinkling of paprika and sprigs of parsley.

Note: This recipe can be made without a blender or processor by finely sieving the egg yolk and then beating in the yogurt with an egg beater. But the processor gives the best result.

CHEESE SOUFFLÉ (For occasional use)

Serves 2

Imperial (Metric)	*American*
1 whole egg *and* 1 yolk	1 whole egg *and* 1 yolk
8 fl oz (225ml) milk	1 cupful milk
4 oz (125g) chopped cheese (mild Cheddar)	1 cupful chopped cheese (mild Cheddar)
1 medium-sized cooked and sliced potato	1 medium-sized cooked and sliced potato
Sea salt	Sea salt
Freshly ground black pepper	Freshly ground black pepper

1. Preheat the oven to 375°F/190°C (Gas Mark 5).
2. Place the egg, the yolk, milk and cheese in a liquidizer and blend for a minute or so.
3. Add the sliced potato and seasoning and blend till all the ingredients are reduced to a smooth purée. (Potato is permissible here as it is much less starchy than using flour for thickening.)
4. Divide the mixture into four buttered, individual, oven-proof ramekins or soufflé dishes.
5. Bake for 30 to 35 minutes till golden brown on top, and serve immediately (they flop quickly!). Serve with Top Favourite All-Seasons Salad (page 152).

CREAMED CAULIFLOWER CHEESE

Serves 4

Imperial (Metric)	*American*
1 medium cauliflower	1 medium cauliflower
4 oz (125g) cottage cheese	1 cupful cottage cheese
4 tablespoonsful double cream	4 tablespoonsful heavy cream
2 oz (50g) grated Cheddar cheese	½ cupful grated Cheddar cheese

1. Cut the cauliflower into thin slices and place in a thick-bottomed pan.
2. Add a little water and simmer gently over a lowish heat until the cauliflower is tender but not mushy and practically no water remains.
3. Using an egg-beater or potato masher beat the cauliflower in the pan to partly cream it.
4. Add the cottage cheese and enough cream to make a creamy mixture.
5. Turn into a shallow, greased baking dish, sprinkle with the grated cheese and brown under the grill.

ALMOND BALLS

Serves 4

Imperial (Metric)	*American*
6 oz (150g) almonds	1½ cupsful almonds
6 oz (150g) additive-free cream cheese	1½ cupsful additive-free cream cheese
A little crushed garlic (optional)	A little crushed garlic (optional)
Toasted sesame seeds	Toasted sesame seeds

1. Skin the almonds by dipping them into hot water to loosen the skins.
2. Chop the almonds and mix with the cream cheese.
3. Add the garlic if liked.
4. Shape the mixture into small balls and roll in the toasted sesame seeds.

Note: This recipe can also be made with finely grated Cheddar cheese in place of the cream cheese, by using a little cream to bind the mixture.

SCRAMBLED TOFU ON AUBERGINE TOASTIES

Serves 4

Imperial (Metric)	*American*
1 pack firm tofu (usually 10.5 oz (297g))	1 pack firm tofu
1 dessertspoon chopped tarragon *or* chopped fresh chives	1 dessertspoon chopped tarragon *or* chopped fresh chives
2 large aubergines	2 large eggplants
2-3 teaspoons olive oil	2-3 teaspoons olive oil
Sesame salt and black pepper	Sesame salt and black pepper
2 teaspoons shoyu	2 teaspoons shoyu

1. Using a blender or food processor, blend the tofu with the chopped herbs and set aside.
2. Slice the aubergines lengthways to allow two slices per person.
3. Brush lightly with olive oil and season with a little freshly ground black pepper.
4. Place under the grill and 'toast' lightly on both sides; keep warm.
5. Heat 2 teaspoons oil gently in frying pan.
6. Pour tofu mixture into the pan and cook for about 5 minutes, stirring constantly.
7. Add shoyu and season to taste.
8. Serve on the toasted aubergine slices.

This makes a quick protein snack which can be varied by flavouring the tofu with whatever fresh herbs are available in season. The first leaves of lovage in the spring are particularly delicious.

WHEATGERM STUFFING

Can be used instead of the usual bread stuffings with roast chicken or turkey, or for stuffing potatoes or beef olives.

Imperial (Metric)	*American*
4 heaped tablespoonsful wheatgerm	4 heaped tablespoonsful wheatgerm
2 tablespoonsful chopped parsley	2 tablespoonsful chopped parsley
1 largish flat mushroom, finely chopped	1 largish flat mushroom, finely chopped
1 tablespoonful sunflower seed oil *or* melted butter	1 tablespoonful sunflower seed oil *or* melted butter
1 egg yolk	1 egg yolk
1 small onion, finely chopped	1 small onion, finely chopped
1 teaspoonful lemon juice	1 teaspoonful lemon juice
1 heaped teaspoonful dried thyme (*or* 2 teaspoonsful fresh thyme)	1 heaped teaspoonful dried thyme (*or* 2 teaspoonsful fresh thyme)
Pinch of dried marjoram	Pinch of dried marjoram
Freshly grated nutmeg	Freshly grated nutmeg
Sea salt	Sea salt
Freshly ground black pepper	Freshly ground black pepper
Water, *or* dry red or white wine, to mix	Water, *or* dry red or white wine, to mix

1. Mix together wheatgerm, parsley, chopped mushroom, oil, egg yolk, onion and lemon juice.
2. Add the herbs and a moderate grating of nutmeg.
3. Season and moisten with water or wine, as necessary.

FRUITY STUFFING

An excellent stuffing for chicken, lamb or pork.

Imperial (Metric)	*American*
3 oz (75g) very sweet dried apricots	½ cupful very sweet dried apricots
4 oz (100g) prunes	¾ cupful prunes
1 large Bramley apple	1 large Bramley apple
3 tablespoonsful wheatgerm	3 tablespoonsful wheatgerm
2 oz (50g) freshly shelled walnuts, or other nuts of choice	½ cupful freshly shelled English walnuts, or other nuts of choice
Juice and grated rind of a well-scrubbed lemon	Juice and grated rind of a well-scrubbed lemon
1 tablespoonful cold pressed sunflower seed oil	1 tablespoonful cold pressed sunflower seed oil
Yolk of 1 egg	Yolk of 1 egg
Sea salt	Sea salt
Freshly ground black pepper	Freshly ground black pepper

1. Blanch the apricots and prunes and soak overnight.
2. Cut up apricots and prunes into small pieces.
3. Peel the apple and chop it coarsely.
4. Chop nuts, also rather coarsely.
5. Put all the ingredients into a mixing bowl and mix together very thoroughly.

GRAVIES AND THICKENINGS WITHOUT FLOUR

To Thicken Gravies:
Use potato flour — this is permissible as so little is required; one teaspoonful or less is often sufficient. Mix 1 teaspoonful potato flour with a little cold water and stir in the meat juices and vegetable stock. Cook at a low heat as a too high heat makes the gravy go thin again.

To Thicken Stews:
Cook the stew with plenty of vegetables and not too much water. When cooked, put some of the liquid from the stew or casserole with some of the vegetables into a liquidizer and blend until nicely thickened.

To Make a Coating Sauce for Vegetables:
Mix an egg yolk into 2 tablespoonsful or more of double/heavy cream, season and add to the remaining vegetable juices in the pan in which the vegetables have been cooked (this should be reduced to 2-3 table-spoonsful) and cook gently over a low heat to avoid curdling. This coating is particularly good for carrots, courgettes (zucchini), french (snap) and runner (green) beans. It not only enhances the taste of the vegetables but makes use of the nutrient-rich vegetable water which is usually thrown away — unless, of course, the vegetables have been steamed.

11.

VEGETABLES

RATATOUILLE

Imperial (Metric)	American
2 large onions	2 large onions
¼ pint (150ml) cold pressed olive oil	⅔ cupful cold pressed olive oil
2 aubergines	2 eggplants
2 red or green peppers	2 red or green peppers
4-6 tomatoes	4-6 tomatoes

1. Peel the onions and slice.
2. Put onions with the oil into a large, thick-bottomed pan over a gentle heat.
3. While the onions are softening cut the unpeeled auber-gines (eggplants) into cubes; remove seeds from the peppers and slice.
4. When the onions are soft, add the aubergines (eggplants) and peppers and allow to stew in the oil very gently for 10 minutes.
5. Peel and slice the tomatoes and add to the rest of veg-etables. Continue to simmer with the lid on the pan for 30 minutes.
6. Take lid off the pan and allow to simmer for a further 10 minutes.

Note: This is a very flexible dish and quantities can be varied according to the availability of the ingredients. Courgettes (zucchini) can be substituted for the peppers if preferred, or if you have a glut in the garden.

COURGETTES DE LUXE

Serves 4

Imperial (Metric)	*American*
8 medium courgettes	8 medium zucchini
Sea salt	Sea salt
3-4 tablespoonsful double cream	3-4 tablespoonsful heavy cream
Freshly ground black pepper	Freshly ground black pepper
Finely chopped parsley	Finely chopped parsley

1. Wash the courgettes (zucchini) and slice into pieces ½-inch (1cm) thick.
2. Pour into a heavy-bottomed pan just sufficient water to cover the bottom of the pan.
3. Add a pinch of salt and the courgettes (zucchini) and cook on a moderate heat for 2 to 3 minutes, stirring constantly, until the skins become a bright green.
4. Cover the pan and turn down to very low, adding a little extra water if necessary.
5. Simmer gently for about 6 minutes until the courgettes (zucchini) are tender but not mushy, stirring occasionally.
6. Remove from heat and add the cream and a sprinkling of black pepper.
7. Leave for a couple of minutes before serving, to allow the cream to thicken slightly and coat the courgettes (zucchini).
8. Turn into a warm serving dish and garnish with chopped parsley.

Note: Using cream in this way is less fatty than the orthodox way of frying or sautéeing courgettes (zucchini) in butter or oil which allows them to soak up an enormous quantity of fat in the cooking process.

PURPLE SPROUTING BROCCOLI WITH LEEKS

Serves 4

Imperial (Metric)

1 lb (450g) purple
  sprouting broccoli
2 large leeks
½ teaspoonful coriander
  seeds
Sea salt
Freshly ground black
  pepper
2 tablespoonsful virgin
  olive oil

American

1 pound purple sprouting
  broccoli
2 large leeks
½ teaspoonful coriander
  seeds
Sea salt
Freshly ground black
  pepper
2 tablespoonsful virgin
  olive oil

1. Wash the broccoli and remove any tough stems and coarse
   or damaged leaves.
2. Steam the broccoli over boiling water until the stalks are
   just tender.
3. Wash and trim the leeks and cut across into slices.
4. Place in a pan containing 1-2 inches (3-5cm) boiling water
   to which you have added a little salt and the crushed
   coriander seeds.
5. Simmer gently for 4-5 minutes.
6. Remove leeks from the water as soon as they are tender,
   drain and place on a warmed serving dish.
7. Remove broccoli from steamer and arrange over the sliced
   leeks.
8. Dress with salt, fresh ground black pepper and pour over
   the olive oil.
9. Serve hot or cold.

CELERIAC PURÉE

Serves 4

Celeriac, or celery root, is a most useful vegetable and can be used to replace potatoes if you want a more substantial root vegetable to accompany meat or chicken dishes.

Imperial (Metric)	*American*
1½ lb (650g) celeriac	1½ pound celeriac
¼ pint (150ml) single cream	⅔ cupful light cream
Sea salt	Sea salt
Freshly ground black pepper	Freshly ground black pepper

1. Peel the celeriac as thinly as possible, cut into even-sized pieces and boil in lightly salted water until tender.
2. Drain the celeriac and pass through a mouli-légumes, or mash by hand or in a food processor.
3. Return the celeriac to the pan over a very low heat. Add the cream slowly, beating it into the purée thoroughly.
4. Season with sea salt (if needed) and freshly ground black pepper.

Note: This purée can also be served as a main course if topped with 4 oz (100g/1 cupful) grated Cheddar cheese and placed under a hot grill for a few minutes.

Parsnips can be prepared in the same way if celeriac is not available.

BUTTERED CABBAGE

Serves 4

Imperial (Metric)	*American*
1 medium-sized firm cabbage	1 medium-sized firm cabbage
Sea salt	Sea salt
½ oz (15g) butter	1 tablespoonful butter
Freshly grated nutmeg	Freshly grated nutmeg
Freshly ground black pepper	Freshly ground black pepper

1. Wash and shred the cabbage.
2. Put ¾-inch (2cm) water into a thick-bottomed pan, add a pinch of salt and bring to the boil.
3. Add the shredded outer leaves of the cabbage, cover pan and boil for 3 minutes.
4. Add the rest of the cabbage and boil until the cabbage is cooked but still crisp (not more than 5 minutes).
5. Drain the cabbage, keeping the water for vegetable stock.
6. Rinse the pan, put in the butter and melt over a medium heat.
7. Put in the cabbage with plenty of freshly ground black pepper and a little nutmeg.
8. Cover pan and allow contents to heat over a low heat for a minute or so, shaking or stirring the contents to mix them thoroughly. Serve at once so that the cabbage retains its crispness and nutty flavour.

SAVOURY MUSHROOMS

Serves 4

Imperial (Metric)	*American*
12 medium to large, nicely cupped mushrooms	12 medium to large, nicely cupped mushrooms
1 oz (25g) butter	2 tablespoonsful butter
Sea salt	Sea salt
Freshly ground black pepper	Freshly ground black pepper
Grated nutmeg	Grated nutmeg

1. Preheat oven to 375°F/190°C (Gas Mark 5).
2. Wash and dry the mushrooms and place them, cup uppermost, in a lightly-buttered fireproof dish.
3. Put a nut of butter into each cup.
4. Sprinkle each with a little salt, black pepper and (most important) a little grated nutmeg.
5. Bake until well cooked; about 20 minutes.

Note: This is a most delicious way of cooking mushrooms and makes commercials ones taste almost like field mushrooms.

GARDENER'S FRENCH BEANS

Imperial (Metric)	*American*
1 lb (450g) very small, young French beans	1 pound very small, young snap beans
1 tablespoonful lemon juice	1 tablespoonful lemon juice
4 tablespoonsful double cream	4 tablespoonsful heavy cream
2 tablespoonsful finely chopped parsley	2 tablespoonsful finely chopped parsley

1. Wash the beans and trim, if necessary; as they should be tiny they will not need stringing or cutting.
2. Place in the top of a steamer and cook over boiling water until they are just tender.
3. Transfer beans to a thick-bottomed pan over a medium heat.
4. Add the lemon juice and cream and stir gently so that the beans are nicely coated.
5. Transfer to a warmed serving dish and sprinkle with chopped parsley.
6. Serve at once.

BUTTERED VEGETABLE SPAGHETTI

Serves 4

Vegetable spaghetti (noodle squash) must surely be one of nature's greatest convenience foods. One plant will provide enough vegetable spaghetti (noodle squash) to feed a family, so it is well worth giving up a corner of the garden to this unusual member of the marrow (squash) family. When sliced, the inside flesh resembles threads of spaghetti — hence its name.

Imperial (Metric)	*American*
1 medium vegetable spaghetti	1 medium noodle squash
2 oz (50g) butter	4 tablespoonsful butter
Sea salt	Sea salt
Freshly ground black pepper	Freshly ground black pepper

1. Wash the vegetable spaghetti (squash) and prick the skin with a fork in two or three places.
2. Place in a steamer and steam over boiling water for about 45 minutes or until the flesh feels tender when pierced with a fork.
3. Remove from the steamer and place on a dish to drain it.
4. Cut the vegetable spaghetti (squash) across into four thick slices and allow any water to drain away.
5. Place the slices on a warmed serving dish, season with a little salt and freshly ground black pepper and place a nut of butter on each slice.
6. Serve at once.

Note: This recipe is for a side dish but vegetable spaghetti (squash) can be served as a main dish for two people if steamed as above, cut in half lengthways and each slice topped with 2 oz (50g/½ cupful) grated Cheddar cheese. Finish by browning under a hot grill.

12.

DESSERTS

FRUIT AND RASPBERRY DESSERT

For festive occasions

Serves 4-6

Imperial (Metric)	American
8 oz (225g) frozen raspberries	8 ounces frozen raspberries
4 large oranges	4 large oranges
8 very sweet dried apricots, previously soaked overnight	8 very sweet dried apricots, previously soaked overnight
4 large ripe pears	4 large ripe pears
4 oz (100g) sweet grapes	⅔ cupful sweet grapes
2-3 kiwi fruits	2-3 kiwi fruits
1 well-ripened banana	1 well-ripened banana

1. Defrost the raspberries and push through a fine nylon sieve.
2. Put the raspberry purée into a large mixing bowl with the juice of 2 of the oranges and some of the juice from the soaked apricots, so that the mixture has a creamy consistency, but is not thin.
3. Prepare the remaining fruit: skin the remaining oranges with a very sharp knife, removing the inner white pith along with the peel — the orange sections can then be removed whole and free of pith; cut the apricots into strips; peel, core and slice one kiwi carefully and cut in thin slices; peel the banana and cut in slices.

4. Mix the prepared fruit into the raspberry sauce.
5. Turn the mixture into a suitable glass dish. Skin the remaining kiwis and cut carefully into thin rings. Mix the small end sections into the fruit mixture. Then arrange the kiwi rings in an overlapping circle on top of the dessert. This gives the dish an exotic appearance.
6. For a finishing touch, arrange a (clean!) half-opened pink rosebud, upright, in the centre, or any other suitable flower in season.

Note: The raspberry purée gives this dessert a beautiful colour and delicious flavour. If the fruits are as sweet as they ought to be, no extra sweetening is necessary. When kiwis are not obtainable, a small handful of sun-dried raisins can be used instead, as a decoration.

Whipped cream can be served separately, if desired, but is not necessary.

FROZEN STRAWBERRY MOUSSE

Serves 4

Imperial (Metric)	*American*
8 oz (225g) defrosted frozen strawberries, *or* fresh ones in season	2 cupsful defrosted frozen strawberries, *or* fresh ones in season
2 tablespoonsful Acacia flower honey, *or* similar mild flavoured honey	2 tablespoonsful Acacia flower honey, *or* similar mild flavored honey
¼ pint (150ml) double cream	⅔ cupful heavy cream
2 rounded tablespoonsful spray-dried skimmed milk powder, dissolved in a very little water	2 rounded tablespoonsful spray-dried skimmed milk powder, dissolved in a very little water

1. Place the strawberries and honey in a liquidizer or food processor and blend to a purée.
2. Whip the cream and dissolved milk powder until it stands in soft peaks.
3. Fold the strawberry purée into the cream.
4. Place in suitable container or individual pots, cover with foil and freeze.

Note: This makes a delicious and very refreshing pudding for occasional use.

SPICED APPLE AND RAISIN PUDDING

Serves 2-3

Imperial (Metric)	*American*
1 lb (450g) sweet dessert apples	1 pound sweet dessert apples
8 oz (225g) cooking apples	8 ounces cooking apples
¾ teaspoonful ground cloves	¾ teaspoonful ground cloves
½ teaspoonful ground cinnamon	½ teaspoonful ground cinnamon
4 oz (100g) raisins	⅔ cupful raisins
¼ whole nutmeg, grated	¼ whole nutmeg, grated
1 tablespoon water	1 tablespoon water

1. Core and peel the apples and slice thinly into a saucepan, adding the spices and raisins.
2. Sprinkle in the water and cook gently, with the lid on, for 10 minutes until the apples are soft and fluffy.
3. Serve either hot or cold (but it is especially good hot on a cold day, and a change from fresh, uncooked fruit).

Note: Made in batches of 3 pounds (1.5 kilos), this is an excellent way of using up windfalls and storing in the deep freeze.

By using mainly sweet dessert apples, it should not be necessary to add sweetening.

THREE QUICK APPLE PUDDINGS

BAKED STUFFED APPLES

1. Wash and core one large eating apple for each person.
2. Fill the centre of each apple with raisins or chopped dates. Place a small teaspoonful of honey over the filling.
3. Place in a baking dish and bake in a moderate oven, 350°F/180°C (Gas Mark 4) until the apples are tender — approximately 35-45 minutes.

APRICOT AND APPLE FOOL

Quantities can be varied according to the number of servings required.

1. Add one-third soaked, dried apricots to two-thirds cooked eating apples.
2. Place in blender or food processor and blend to a thick, but not too fine, purée.
3. Add a little honey to taste and serve decorated with whipped cream and a sprinkling of chopped nuts.

APPLE AND RAISIN PUDDING

1. Place peeled and sliced eating apples, interlaced with raisins, in a baking dish and pour over the juice of one orange diluted with a little water.
2. Bake in a moderate oven, 350°F/180°C (Gas Mark 4) until soft.
3. Sprinkle with a mixture of crushed nuts and wheatgerm and serve with whipped cream. Good either hot or cold.

APRICOT MOUSSE

Serves 4

Imperial (Metric)	*American*
8 oz (225g) dried apricots	1½ cupsful dried apricots
4 tablespoonsful natural yogurt	4 tablespoonsful natural yogurt
Flaked almonds for topping	Slivered almonds for topping

1. Wash and blanch the dried apricots and soak overnight in just enough water to cover them.
2. Place the apricots, with their juice, in a liquidizer and blend until smooth.
3. Fold the yogurt into the apricot purée and pour into individual glasses.
4. Decorate with a topping of almonds.

Variation:
For a richer dessert for special occasions, fold in ¼ pint (150ml/⅔ cupful) whipped cream before pouring into the glasses.

NECTARINES IN A GLASS

Serves 4

Imperial (Metric)	*American*
4 really ripe nectarines	4 really ripe nectarines
4 teaspoonsful mild clear honey, such as Acacia	4 teaspoonsful mild clear honey, such as Acacia
White wine, not too dry	White wine, not too dry

1. Wash the nectarines well and dry carefully so that the skin is not damaged.
2. Do not peel them but, using a stainless steel knife, slice each one straight into a wine goblet. (To get the best effect make the first incision down the natural division of the fruit from stalk to flower end. Slice out one section and continue slicing, turning the fruit as you cut until all you have left is the stone.)
3. Dribble 1 teaspoonful of honey over each sliced nectarine and top up each glass with white wine.

Note: Do not prepare too long in advance of the meal or the fruit may become sodden.

Peaches may be prepared in the same way but they should be peeled. In France, red wine is usually used to cover the peaches.

CHRISTMAS PUDDING

This is a favourite recipe with family and friends. it contains no flour or sugar and does not produce the 'distended' feeling usually experienced after eating the orthodox Christmas Plum Pudding.

Imperial (Metric)

8 oz (225g) sultanas (whole)

8 oz (225g) sultanas (minced)

8 oz (225g) large seeded raisins (minced)

3 oz (75g) seeded raisins (whole)

16 Santa Clara prunes, soaked for 2 days until soft, then stoned and minced

4 oz (100g) finely chopped walnuts and almonds

8 fl oz (225ml) prune juice (from soaking prunes)

Juice of 1 large orange (and some grated rind if oranges are organically grown and therefore unsprayed)

8 oz (225g) ground almonds or freshly ground hazelnuts

4 fl oz (125ml) brandy or whisky

2 egg yolks, well beaten

American

1¾ cupsful golden seedless raisins (whole)

1¾ cupsful golden seedless raisins (minced)

1¾ cupsful large seeded raisins (minced)

½ cupful seeded raisins (whole)

16 Santa Clara prunes, soaked for 2 days until soft, then stoned and minced

¾ cupful finely chopped English walnuts and almonds

1 cupful prune juice (from soaking prunes)

Juice of 1 large orange (and some grated rind if oranges are organically grown and therefore unsprayed)

2 cupsful ground almonds or freshly ground hazelnuts

½ cupful brandy or whisky

2 egg yolks, well beaten

1. Place all the ingredients in a mixing bowl and mix well together.
2. Grease a 2¼ pint (1.25 litre/6 cup) pudding basin and transfer mixture into it.
3. Cover the top with buttered greaseproof paper and an outer covering of foil.
4. Steam gently for 1 hour.
5. To serve, turn out carefully onto a warm serving dish, decorate with a piece of berried holly, pour a little brandy over the pudding and set alight.
6. Can be accompanied with whipped cream, flavoured with brandy.

Note: This pudding has a rich, fruity flavour but if you prefer the traditional spicy flavour of Christmas pudding one teaspoonful of ground mixed spice can be added to the mixture.

Freezing: This pudding will freeze satisfactorily for six weeks. Allow to thaw out gradually and steam for 45 minutes.

YOGURT

Homemade yogurt is quick and easy to make. You need no special equipment apart from a wide-necked vacuum flask (also useful for transporting soup for packed lunches) and a dairy thermometer. If your family likes yogurt you will save pounds every year by making your own.

Imperial (Metric)	*American*
1 pint (550ml) milk (full cream *or* skimmed)	2½ cupsful milk (full cream *or* skimmed)
1 tablespoonful spray-dried skimmed milk powder (optional)	1 tablespoonful spray-dried skimmed milk powder (optional)
1 teaspoonful natural yogurt (as starter)	1 teaspoonful natural yogurt (as starter)

1. Put the milk into a thick-bottomed pan.
2. Whisk in the milk powder if liked; it gives a better texture and thicker yogurt.
3. Heat the milk to 180°F/82°C or to just below boiling point.
4. Cool the milk, by placing the pan in a sink of cold water, to 110°F/43°C.
5. Rinse out the vacuum flask with hot water. Pour most of the milk into the vacuum flask.
6. Blend 1 teaspoonful of natural yogurt with the remaining milk and add to the vacuum flask.
7. Put the lid on firmly and shake to mix well.
8. Leave for 4-6 hours or until firm curd is obtained.
9. Remove the stopper and put flask in refrigerator to cool and firm the yogurt.
10. You can use 1 teaspoonful of this yogurt to 'start' the next batch, but you will need to revert to a starter of fresh 'live' yogurt every 7-10 batches.

Note: Other methods of incubation (excluding commercial yogurt makers) are:

1. Put the prepared milk into a *Tupperware* (or similar) fluid container.

2. Place the container in box surrounded by polystyrene chips (the kind used for packing), *or*
3. Wrap the container in a warm blanket and leave in a warm place, such as the airing cupboard or on a rack over a solid fuel cooker.

Once made, the yogurt can be used in all the usual ways. For fruit yogurt, mix in the prepared fruit only *after* the yogurt has been made.

The following recipe for pineapple yogurt makes a quick and delicious dessert to follow a protein main course.

PINEAPPLE YOGURT

Mix fresh, crushed, unsweetened pineapple with plain yogurt as desired. Serve in individual glasses and sprinkle with sunflower seeds.

DINNER PARTY ICE CREAM

Imperial (Metric)	*American*
½ pint (275ml) double cream	1⅓ cupsful heavy cream
½ pint (275 ml) single cream	1⅓ cupsful light cream
1 level tablespoonful spray-dried milk powder	1 level tablespoonful spray-dried milk powder
A little cold milk	1¾ cupsful chopped raisins
8 oz (225g) chopped raisins	1¾ cupsful chopped cashews or other nuts
8 oz (225g) chopped cashews or other nuts	1 tablespoonful maple syrup
1 tablespoonful maple syrup	2 teaspoonsful honey
1 dessertspoonful honey	

1. Mix the creams together and whisk until thick.
2. Mix the dried milk to a creamy consistency with a little cold milk and stir into the whipped cream.
3. Add the maple syrup and honey to sweeten, and the chopped raisins and nuts.
4. Place in suitable container, cover with foil and freeze. Stir once during freezing.

Note: The addition of the dried milk powder is the secret of the success of this recipe; it prevents the ice cream becoming hard and icy and ensures a professional smoothness of texture. It will keep this texture even if kept in the freezer for a week or longer.

APRICOT SAUCE

Imperial (Metric)

8 oz (225g) sweet dried
 apricots
Juice of 1 large, fresh
 orange *or* diluted frozen
 unsweetened orange
 juice

American

1½ cupsful sweet dried
 apricots
Juice of 1 large, fresh
 orange *or* diluted frozen
 unsweetened orange
 juice

1. Wash the apricots (blanch in boiling water and rinse again
   if apricots are not organically grown).
2. Prepare the apricots by covering with boiling water and
   leaving to soak overnight.
3. Next day place the apricots and some of the juice from
   soaking them in a blender with enough orange juice to
   make a sauce of medium thickness. It is difficult to be
   precise about quantities but if you run the motor at low
   speed you can add more orange juice if required until the
   sauce has reached the right consistency.
4. Serve as a dressing for peeled and sliced pears or other
   fruit. A little whipping or double cream makes a delicious
   addition to the sauce, giving it a smoother texture.

SUGGESTIONS FOR PACKED MEALS

There is no need always to think of packed meals in terms of bread sandwiches. A protein meal is just as easy to transport.

A 'bagged' meal can consist of slices of cold meat, or chicken left over from Sunday lunch placed between lettuce leaves, or a chunk of cheese with a selection from celery sticks, raw carrots, slices of fresh fennel root, cress, tomatoes, cucumber chunks, green or red pepper rings or chunks of fresh coconut. To finish, pack any of the acid fruits such apples, pears and oranges. If still hungry, sunflower seeds make a delicious filler and on cold days the meal can be preceded by a hot vegetable soup carried in a thermos.

Another good packed meal consists of individual cold omelettes (page 180) accompanied by lettuce, cress or other salad vegetables followed by fresh fruit.

PART FOUR
RECIPES FOR STARCH MEALS

13.

SOUPS

CELERIAC SOUP

Serves 4-6

Imperial (Metric)	*American*
1 onion	1 onion
2 celeriac, weighing in total about 1½ lbs (700g)	2 celeriac, weighing in total about 1½ pounds
2 oz (50g) butter	4 tablespoonsful butter
1½ pints (850ml) vegetable stock	3¾ cupsful vegetable stock
Sea salt	Sea salt
Freshly ground black pepper	Freshly ground black pepper
4 tablespoonsful single cream	4 tablespoonsful light cream
Chopped fresh parsley	Chopped fresh parsley

1. Peel and chop the onion, peel the celeriac and cut into cubes.
2. Melt the butter in a heavy saucepan and cook the onions gently for 2-3 minutes. Add the celeriac and cook for a further 5 minutes, stirring constantly.
3. Add the stock, bring to the boil, cover pan and simmer until celeriac is tender.
4. Pour into a liquidizer and blend until smooth.
5. Return to the pan, add seasoning and reheat.
6. Stir in the cream and serve with plenty of chopped parsley.

POTATO SOUP

Serves 4

Imperial (Metric)	*American*
1 leek	1 leek
1 oz (25g) butter	2 tablespoonsful butter
4 potatoes weighing between 6-8 oz (150-225g) each	4 potatoes weighing between 6-8 ounces each
1 pint (550ml) vegetable stock *or* water flavoured with ½ teaspoonful yeast extract	2½ cupsful vegetable stock *or* water flavored with ½ teaspoonful yeast extract
Sea salt	Sea salt
Freshly ground black pepper	Freshly ground black pepper
Grated nutmeg *or* 1 teaspoonful curry powder	Grated nutmeg *or* 1 teaspoonsful curry powder

1. Wash the leek thoroughly and slice.
2. Melt the butter in a thick-bottomed pan and add the chopped leek. Allow to cook gently without colouring.
3. Add the potatoes, scraped and quartered, and the vegetable stock.
4. Bring to the boil, cover the pan and simmer gently until potatoes are tender.
5. Place in a liquidizer and blend until smooth.
6. Return to the pan, season with salt and pepper and add a little milk to give a creamier consistency (or more stock if preferred).
7. Lastly add a pinch of nutmeg *or* a teaspoonful of curry powder.
8. Reheat and serve sprinkled with chopped parsley.

MIXED VEGETABLE SOUP

Serves 4-6

Imperial (Metric)	*American*
8 oz (225g) parsnips	8 ounces parsnips
8 oz (225g) carrots	8 ounces carrots
8 oz (225g) swedes or turnips	8 ounces of rutabaga or turnips
2 sticks celery	2 stalks celery
2 oz (50g) butter	4 tablespoonsful butter
2 pints (1 litre) vegetable stock	5 cupsful vegetable stock
1 teaspoonful yeast extract	1 teaspoonful yeast extract
Sea salt	Sea salt
Freshly ground black pepper	Freshly ground black pepper
Freshly chopped parsley	Freshly chopped parsley

1. Cut all the root vegetables into smallish slices and chop the celery.
2. Melt the butter in a heavy pan, add the root vegetables and cook them gently for about 5 minutes.
3. Add the vegetable stock, yeast extract and chopped celery and bring to the boil. Turn down heat and simmer gently for about 10 minutes until the vegetables are tender but not mushy.
4. Place in a liquidizer and blend for a few seconds so that the texture is thick but still fairly coarse.
5. Return to the pan and reheat; season with salt and pepper.
6. Serve with a good sprinkling of chopped parsley.

Note: If you grow herbs and have a lovage plant, the addition of *one* leaf of lovage improves the flavour of this soup.

ASPARAGUS SOUP

This soup can be made from the trimmings from a bundle of asparagus — the tips being served as a vegetable in the usual way.

Serves 4

Imperial (Metric)	*American*
trimmings from a 2 lb (1 kilo) bundle of asparagus	Trimmings from a 2 pound bundle of asparagus
4 oz (125g) chopped onion	1½ cupsful chopped onion
1½ oz (40g) butter	3 tablespoonsful butter
1 dessertspoonful potato flour	2 teaspoonsful potato flour
¾ pint (½ litre) asparagus stock (from cooking tips and trimmings)	2 cupsful asparagus stock (from cooking tips and trimmings)
Sea salt	Sea salt
Freshly ground black pepper	Freshly ground black pepper
1 tablespoon chopped parsley	1 tablespoonful chopped parsley
2 tablespoonsful double cream	2 tablespoonsful heavy cream

1. Cook the asparagus bundle in the usual way. Serve the tips as a vegetable. Reserve the trimmings and the asparagus liquor.
2. In a thick-bottomed pan, melt the butter, add the chopped onion and cook gently until the onion is golden.
3. Add the asparagus trimmings and liquor and simmer for about 10 minutes to extract the full flavour.
4. Purée the liquid in a blender and pass through a sieve to remove any stringy pieces.
5. Return to pan and add the potato flour which has been mixed to a smooth paste with a little water.
6. Add seasoning to taste and heat until just below boiling point.
7. Add parsley, stir in cream and serve.

14.

SALADS

POTATO SALAD

Serves 4

Imperial (Metric)	*American*
4 large *or* 8 small new potatoes	4 large *or* 8 small new potatoes
2 sticks of celery	2 stalks of celery
2-3 spring onions	2-3 scallions
2 tablespoonsful single cream	2 tablespoonsful light cream
Sea salt	Sea salt
Freshly ground black pepper	Freshly ground black pepper
3-4 mint leaves	3-4 fresh mint leaves

1. Cook the potatoes in their skins.
2. While still warm remove the skins and leave to cool.
3. Dice the potatoes, chop the celery and spring onions (scallions) and mix together.
4. Dress with the cream seasoned with salt and pepper and flavoured with chopped mint leaves.

Note: Left-over waxy potatoes can also be used to make this salad.

BROWN RICE SALAD

Serves 4

Imperial (Metric)	*American*
8 oz (225g) long grain brown rice	1 cupful long grain brown rice
1¼ pints (700ml) water	3 cupsful water
1 level teaspoonful sea salt	1 level teaspoonful sea salt
3 spring onions, chopped finely	3 scallions, chopped finely
1 red pepper, de-seeded and sliced finely	1 red pepper, de-seeded and sliced finely
2 oz (50g) seedless raisins	½ cupful seedless raisins
2 oz (50g) pecan nuts, coarsely chopped	½ cupful coarsely chopped pecan nuts
1 tablespoonful olive oil	1 tablespoonful olive oil
Salt and freshly ground black pepper to taste	Salt and freshly ground black pepper to taste
A little chopped fresh parsley	A little chopped fresh parsley

1. Put the rice into a sieve and pour cold water through it to remove any dirt.
2. Put the rice and water into a large pan and bring to the boil.
3. Allow to boil for 1 minute, put lid on the pan and turn heat right down so that the water is barely at simmering point.
4. Leave to cook for about 40 minutes, then test. The grains should be chewy, not mushy.
5. Drain the rice into a colander and rinse with cold water. Set aside until cool.
6. While the rice is cooking and cooling, prepare the remaining ingredients.
7. When the rice is almost cold add the onions, pepper, raisins and nuts.
8. Pour oil over the salad and toss well together, adjusting seasoning if necessary.
9. Place the salad in a serving dish and garnish with chopped parsley.

TABBOULEH

Serves 6

Imperial (Metric)	*American*
8 oz (225g) bulghur (cracked wheat)	1 cupful bulghur (cracked wheat)
3 tablespoonsful finely chopped spring onions *or* 1 onion, finely chopped	3 tablespoonsful finely chopped scallions *or* 1 onion, finely chopped
Salt and freshly milled black pepper	Salt and freshly milled black pepper
6 tablespoonsful finely chopped parsley	6 tablespoonsful finely chopped parsley
3 tablespoonsful finely chopped fresh mint	3 tablespoonsful finely chopped fresh mint
4 tablespoonsful olive oil	4 tablespoonsful olive oil
2 tablespoonsful grated lemon rind	2 tablespoonsful grated lemon rind
Lettuce	Lettuce
1 green pepper	1 green pepper

1. Soak the bulghur in water for about ½ hour. Drain and squeeze out as much moisture as you can with your hands. Spread out on absorbent kitchen paper to dry still further.
2. Mix the bulghur with the chopped onion, turning thoroughly to allow the juices to penetrate the grains. Season to taste with salt and pepper.
3. Add the parsley, mint, olive oil, lemon rind and mix well. Taste to find out whether more seasoning or lemon is needed. There should be a distinct lemony flavour.
4. Pile onto a large serving dish lined with crisp lettuce leaves and strips of green pepper.

PECAN AND PASTA SALAD

Serves 4

Imperial (Metric)	*American*
4 oz (100g) wholemeal pasta shells	2 cupsful wholewheat pasta shells
1 green pepper, de-seeded	1 green pepper, de-seeded
4 oz (100g) pecan nuts	¾ cupful pecan nuts
2 oz (50g) raisins	⅓ cupful raisins
4 tablespoonsful soured cream dressing for starch meals (page 226)	4 tablespoonsful soured cream dressing for starch meals (page 226)

1. Cook pasta in boiling salted water until just tender.
2. Drain well and allow to cool.
3. Chop the green pepper finely and mix with pasta.
4. Add pecan nuts and raisins.
5. Mix well with the soured cream dressing and serve.

Note: This salad is substantial enough to be served as a main dish. If used as a side dish, the portions should be smaller and this quantity would serve 6-8.

BROAD BEAN AND SAVORY SALAD

Serves 4

Imperial (Metric)	*American*
2 lb (900g) young tender broad beans	2 pounds young tender Windsor beans
2-3 sprigs of summer savory	2-3 sprigs summer savory
Mustard and cress	Mustard and cress
¼ pint (150ml) soured cream	⅔ cupful soured cream
Sea salt	Sea salt
Paprika	Paprika

1. If the bean pods are really small and tender simply wash, top and tail them and cut into short lengths. If larger, shell the beans.
2. Put the beans into *just* enough boiling water to cover them, add a pinch of salt and a sprig of savory and cook with the lid on the pan until they are just tender (10-15 minutes).
3. Drain the beans and allow to cool.
4. Arrange on a bed of mustard and cress and dress with the soured cream which has been seasoned with a pinch of paprika and a teaspoonful of finely chopped savory leaves.

CARROT AND RAISIN SALAD

Serves 4

Imperial (Metric)

American

2 oz (50g) seedless raisins
8 oz (225g) grated raw
  carrot
Lettuce
3 tablespoonsful single
  cream
Sea salt
Freshly ground black
  pepper

⅓ cupful seedless raisins
1½ cupsful grated raw
  carrot
Lettuce
3 tablespoonsful light
  cream
Sea salt
Freshly ground black
  pepper

1. Soak the raisins in water for a couple of hours before
   making the salad.
2. Mix the grated carrot with the soaked raisins and arrange
   on a bed of lettuce.
3. Season the cream with salt and pepper and pour over the
   grated carrots.

BANANA AND DATE SALAD

The quantities for this salad will vary according to the number of people to be served.

Imperial (Metric)	*American*
1 small banana per person	1 small banana per person
Grated or very finely chopped nuts *or* toasted sesame seeds	Grated or finely chopped nuts *or* toasted sesame seeds
1 lettuce or other greens	1 lettuce or other greens
4 dates per person	4 dates per person
4 oz (100g) additive-free cream cheese	½ cupful additive-free cream cheese
About ⅓ pint (200ml) single cream	about ¾ cupful light cream
1 teaspoonful clear mild honey such as Acacia	1 teaspoonful clear mild honey such as Acacia
Fresh mint leaves *or* freshly grated rind of a well-scrubbed lemon	Fresh mint leaves *or* freshly grated rind of a well-scrubbed lemon

1. Cut the bananas into quarters and roll the pieces in the grated nuts or toasted sesame seeds.
2. Wash and dry the lettuce leaves and arrange on a serving dish to form a base for the other ingredients.
3. Arrange the banana pieces on the bed of lettuce.
4. Remove stones from the dates, fill the centres with cream cheese and arrange on the dish.
5. Dress the salad with the cream, sweetened with a teaspoonful of honey and flavoured with a pinch of freshly chopped mint leaves or a little grated lemon rind.

AUBERGINE PÂTÉ

Serves 4

Imperial (Metric)	*American*
3 large aubergines	3 large eggplants
1 clove garlic	1 clove garlic
2 tablespoonsful olive oil	2 tablespoonsful olive oil
1 tablespoonful lemon juice*	1 tablespoonful lemon juice*
Sea salt and freshly ground black pepper	Sea salt and freshly ground black pepper
1 dessertspoonful chopped fresh tarragon if available**	2 teaspoonful chopped fresh tarragon if available**

1. Preheat oven to 350°F/180°C (Gas Mark 4).
2. Place the aubergines (eggplants) in a shallow baking dish and bake in the oven for about 45 minutes.
3. Remove aubergines (eggplants) from the oven and allow to cool slightly. Cut in half and remove the flesh; put this through the medium plate of a mouli-légumes or vegetable mill.
4. Add the crushed garlic and stir in the olive oil and enough of the lemon juice to sharpen the purée.
5. Add salt and pepper to taste, stir in the chopped tarragon and put into a dish.
6. Chill thoroughly before serving.
7. Serve on wholewheat toast as a light meal or in smaller quantities as a starter. This will freeze but is better fresh.

*Permissible because so little is used.
**If no tarragon available, decorate the pâté with a little finely chopped parsley before serving.

Salad Dressings for Starch Meals

Non-acid French Dressing:

Use equal parts of fresh raw tomato juice and olive or sunflower seed oil. Season with sea salt, paprika and any fresh herbs available. Fresh chopped tarragon or basil are very good additions.

Simple Cream Dressing:

Add sea salt, freshly ground black pepper and any fresh chopped herbs available to ¼ pint (150ml/⅔ cupful) single (light) cream. Good with mixed shredded raw vegetable salads.

Avocado Cream Dressing:

Blend the flesh of one ripe avocado with a little thin cream and season with sea salt and paprika. Very good with a mixed green salad.

Egg Yolk Topping:

Egg yolks are a rich source of vitamins and minerals. Hard boil the eggs, chop the yolks finely (or press through a sieve) and season lightly with sea salt. Use as a decorative and nutritious topping for salads and vegetable dishes.

Cooked vegetable salads can be dressed simply with a little seasoned olive oil.
The best oil for salads and cooking is cold-pressed virgin olive oil. As this is now so expensive and it is often difficult to obtain a really good tasting one, cold-pressed sesame oil and sunflower seed oil are the best alternatives.

Soured Cream Dressing:

Imperial (Metric)	American
¼ pint (150ml) soured cream	⅔ cupful soured cream
Freshly grated rind of a well-scrubbed lemon	Freshly grated rind of a well-scrubbed lemon
Sea salt	Sea salt
Freshly ground black pepper	Freshly ground black pepper
1 teaspoonful clear, mild honey (optional)	1 teaspoonful clear, mild honey (optional)

1. Mix all ingredients well together before pouring over the salad to be dressed. This dressing is best prepared just before it is required.

15.

MAIN DISHES

SPAGHETTI WITH PESTO

Serves 4

Imperial (Metric)	*American*
8 oz (225g) wholemeal spaghetti	8 ounces wholewheat spaghetti
Sea salt	Sea salt
1 large handful chopped fresh basil	1 large handful chopped fresh basil
4 oz (100g) pistachio nuts *or* pine kernels	¾ cupful pistachio nuts *or* pine kernels
6 large tomatoes	6 large tomatoes
8 tablespoonsful olive oil	8 tablespoonsful olive oil
Black pepper	Black pepper

1. Half fill a large saucepan with water, add a tablespoonful of sea salt and bring water to the boil.
2. Put the spaghetti into the water, pushing it down into the pan as it softens.
3. Simmer gently for about 10 minutes until the spaghetti is just tender but still has a bite to it — 'al denté'.
4. Drain the spaghetti well and slide it into a well oiled and heated dish.
5. While the spaghetti is simmering make the pesto.
6. Peel the tomatoes, chop coarsely and place in a blender.
7. Add basil, nuts, salt and pepper and olive oil.
8. Blend everything together and adjust seasoning if necessary.
9. Pour the pesto over the spaghetti, add a little butter and toss the spaghetti well. Serve at once.

PASTA SHELLS WITH PARSLEY SAUCE

Serves 4

Imperial (Metric)	*American*
8oz (225g) wholemeal pasta shells	2 cupsful wholewheat pasta shells
Sea salt	Sea salt

For the parsley sauce:

Imperial (Metric)	*American*
1 oz (25g) butter	2 tablespoonsful butter
1 oz (25g) wholemeal flour	¼ cupful wholewheat flour
½ pint (275ml) milk	1⅓ cupsful milk
2-3 tablespoonsful chopped parsley	2-3 tablespoonsful chopped parsley
Sea salt	Sea salt
Freshly ground black pepper	Freshly ground black pepper

1. Place the pasta shells in a saucepan of boiling water with a pinch of salt and cook for 10-12 minutes or until *al dente* (just cooked but not soggy).
2. In a thick saucepan melt the butter and stir in the flour. Stir with a wooden spoon until the mixture bubbles.
3. Remove pan from the heat and slowly add the milk stirring all the time to prevent lumps forming.
4. Return to heat and stir constantly until the sauce thickens and has reached boiling point.
5. Wash and chop the parsley and add to the sauce.
6. Drain the pasta and place on a serving dish.
7. Reheat sauce and pour over the pasta. Serve with a green salad.

RICE WITH LEEKS AND CASHEW NUTS

Serves 4

Imperial (Metric)	*American*
8 oz (225g) long grain brown rice	1 cupful long grain brown rice
1¼ pints (700ml) water	3 cupsful water
4 large *or* 6 small leeks	4 large *or* 6 small leeks
1 oz (25g) butter	2 tablespoonsful butter
2 oz (50g) seedless raisins	⅓ cupful seedless raisins
2oz (50g) cashew nuts	⅓ cupful cashew nuts

1. Put the rice and water into a pan (one which has a lid) and bring to the boil; boil fiercely for 5 minutes and then put lid on pan and turn heat right down. Leave for 40 minutes.
2. Put the butter into a thick-bottomed saucepan and melt gently — add the leeks, which have been thoroughly cleaned and cut into thin rounds by slicing across the stems.
3. Cover the pan and turn the heat down so that the leeks cook gently in their own liquid until tender, but still crisp. Be careful not to overcook. The green part of the leek should remain a bright green. 5-10 minutes is usually long enough for this process but the time varies a little according to the thickness of the leeks.
4. When the leeks are done, transfer them to a colander to drain, return to the pan and add the raisins and cashew nuts.
5. When the rice is done mix the contents of the two saucepans together and test for seasoning, adding a little sea salt and ground black pepper if necessary and serve.

RICE PILAFF

Serves 4

Imperial (Metric)	*American*
1 lb (450g) mixed raw vegetables — choose from: peas, carrots, celery, leeks, red or green peppers or celeriac	2 cupsful mixed raw vegetables — choose from: peas, carrots, celery, leeks, red or green peppers or celeriac
1 oz (25g) butter	2 tablespoonsful butter
Dried mixed herbs	Dried mixed herbs
Sea salt	Sea salt
Freshly milled black pepper	Freshly milled black pepper
12 oz (350g) cooked brown rice*	1½ cupsful cooked brown rice*
2 oz (50g) raisins	½ cupful raisins
2 oz (50g) chopped nuts	½ cupful chopped nuts
1 teaspoonful curry powder (optional)	1 teaspoonful curry powder (optional)

1. Prepare the raw vegetables; dice carrots and celery or celeriac. Slice the leeks and peppers.
2. Place the prepared vegetables (except peas) in a heavy stewpan with the butter.
3. Cook gently on a low heat for about 10 minutes, stirring frequently.
4. Add just enough water to cook the vegetables without sticking to the pan, a pinch of dried mixed herbs, salt and pepper. For variety add a teaspoonful or so of curry powder as soon as the carrots are cooked.
5. Cook the peas in a separate pan to retain their colour.
6. When the vegetable mixture is tender and of a thick consistency add the rice, raisins, peas and chopped nuts.

*To Cook Brown Rice

To every 8 oz (225g/1 cupful) brown rice allow 1¼ pints (700ml/3 cupsful) water. Put the rice and water into a thick-bottomed pan (one with a well-fitting lid) and bring to the boil. Boil for 5 minutes, then cover the pan and turn the heat down as low as you can so that the water is barely simmering. Leave for 40 minutes. Do not stir while cooking. When the rice is tender the water should have been completely absorbed but if there should be any left, drain the rice and return to the pan for a few minutes to dry off before serving.

VEGETABLE CASSEROLE

Serves 4

Imperial (Metric)	*American*
1 oz (25g) butter	2 tablespoonsful butter
3 onions, peeled and sliced	3 onions, peeled and sliced
1 lb (450g) carrots, scrubbed and sliced	2½ cupsful scrubbed and sliced carrots
1 lb (450g) potatoes, peeled and sliced	2½ cupsful peeled and sliced potatoes
2 sticks celery, washed and chopped	2 stalks celery, washed and chopped
1 green pepper, washed, de-seeded and cut into strips	1 green pepper, washed, de-seeded and cut into strips
8 oz (225g) button mushrooms, washed and sliced	3 cupsful button mushrooms, washed and sliced
1 pint (575ml) water *or* vegetable stock	2½ cupsful water *or* vegetable stock
1 tablespoonful tomato purée	1 tablespoonful tomato paste
1 large bay leaf	1 large bay leaf
1 dessertspoonful potato flour	2 teaspoonsful potato flour
Sea salt	Sea salt
Freshly ground black pepper	Freshly ground black pepper

1. Preheat oven to 375°F/190°C (Gas Mark 5).
2. Melt butter in heavy frying pan and sauté onions until golden. Add rest of vegetables and continue to cook for a further 2-3 minutes stirring often.
3. Transfer to flameproof casserole dish and add water or stock, tomato purée, bay leaf and seasoning.
4. Bring contents of casserole to boil then transfer to oven and cook for 45 minutes.
5. Remove from oven and add potato flour which has been mixed to a smooth paste with a little water. Stir well, adjust seasoning and return to oven for a further 15 minutes.

HAZELNUT ROAST

Serves 4

Imperial (Metric)	*American*
10 oz (300g) hazelnuts	2 cupsful filberts
8 oz (225g) wholemeal breadcrumbs	4 cupsful wholewheat breadcrumbs
8 oz (225g) chopped onion	1⅓ cupsful\chopped onion
8 oz (225g) grated carrot	1⅓ cupsful grated carrot
Sea salt	Sea salt
Freshly milled black pepper	Freshly milled black pepper
½ teaspoonful dried mixed herbs	½ teaspoonful dried mixed herbs
2 egg yolks	2 egg yolks
A little milk	A little milk

1. Preheat oven to 375°F/190°C (Gas Mark 5).
2. Chop the hazelnuts coarsely.
3. Mix the nuts, breadcrumbs, onion and carrots well together.
4. Add salt and pepper to taste, and the dried herbs.
5. Add the beaten egg yolks and, if necessary, a little milk to bind the mixture.
6. Place in a well greased loaf tin and bake for 45 minutes. Serve with a cooked green vegetable or a green salad.

POTATOES DAUPHINOIS À LA HAY

Serves 2

Imperial (Metric)	*American*
2 baking-sized waxy new season's potatoes (such as Wilja) per person	2 baking-sized waxy new season's potatoes (such as Wilja) per person
1 small onion per person (or adjust quantity according to taste)	1 small onion per person (or adjust quantity according to taste)
Sea salt	Sea salt
Freshly ground black pepper	Freshly ground black pepper
A little double cream *or* about ½ oz (15g) butter	A little heavy cream *or* about 1 tablespoonful butter

1. Scrub the potatoes well to remove outer thin brown skins and cut into thin slices. Preheat the oven to 425°F/220°C (Gas Mark 7).
2. Roughly chop up the onion — quantity according to taste.
3. Place an inch (5mm) or so of water in a thick-bottomed pan, add the chopped onion and sliced potatoes.
4. Season lightly with sea salt and freshly ground black pepper.
5. Cook over moderate heat for about 6 to 8 minutes, until the potatoes are nearly cooked and there is only a little water left in the pan.
6. Turn the contents of the pan, including the valuable potato water, into a shallow buttered fireproof oven dish (*Pyrex* or *Corning Ware*).
7. Arrange the potato slices to make a nice flat surface and just dribble over it some double cream, or dab all over with a piece of butter.
8. Bake for about 30 minutes or until the potato slices on top are golden brown and becoming crisp.

Note: This is an excellent and very savoury main course dish for a starch meal, accompanied with a salad or vegetables, or

just mustard and cress. Cooked this way potatoes are economical with fat (butter or cream) compared to 'Potatoes Anna'
or to baked jacket potatoes which tempt one to overdo the
accompanying butter. (This recipe is now so popular with my
husband that he prefers it to any other way of cooking
potatoes — D.G.)

This dish can also be made with old potatoes, but the skins
will then have to be removed, *as thinly as possible* with a
vegetable peeler.

POTATO AND LEEK HOTPOT

Serves 2

Imperial (Metric)	*American*
2 medium leeks	2 medium leeks
1 oz (25g) butter	2 tablespoonsful butter
1½ lbs (700g) potatoes	1½ pounds potatoes
8 fl oz (225ml) water	1 cupful water
Sea salt	Sea salt
Freshly ground black pepper	Freshly ground black pepper
2 tablespoonsful double cream	2 tablespoonsful heavy cream
Chopped parsley	Chopped parsley

1. Clean and slice the leeks.
2. Melt the butter in a heavy-bottomed pan and add the sliced leeks.
3. Cook on a low heat, stirring frequently until the leeks are a light golden colour.
4. Pare and slice the potatoes and add them, with the water, to the leeks.
5. Cook over very low heat, stirring occasionally, till the potatoes are cooked and almost sticking to the bottom of the pan — this gives the hotpot its excellent flavour! If the mixture becomes at all dry add a little more water.
6. Add the seasoning and stir in the cream just before serving. Sprinkle with chopped parsley for decoration.

JACKET POTATOES WITH MUSHROOM FILLING

Serves 4

Imperial (Metric)	*American*
4 medium King Edward potatoes of uniform shape and sound skins	4 medium potatoes of uniform shape and sound skins
A little sunflower seed oil	A little sunflower seed oil
4 fl oz (125ml) hot milk	½ cupful hot milk
½ oz (15g) butter	1 tablespoonful butter
Sea salt	Sea salt
Freshly ground black pepper	Freshly ground black pepper
Freshly grated nutmeg	Freshly grated nutmeg

1. Preheat oven to 400°F/200°C (Gas Mark 6).
2. Scrub the potatoes well, prick with a fork and smear the skins with sunflower seed oil.
3. Bake in the oven for 1 hour, or until the skins are crisp.
4. Cut potatoes in two, remove flesh and return skins to the oven to keep crisp.
5. Mash the potato flesh well in a saucepan with the milk and butter to make a light creamy mixture.
6. Season to taste with salt, black pepper and especially the nutmeg.
7. Refill the potato shells with the mixture, making a hollow in the centres with the back of a spoon to hold the mushroom filling.

For the Mushroom Filling:

Imperial (Metric)	*American*
8 oz (225g) open, black-gilled mushrooms	4 cupsful open, black-gilled mushrooms
6 tablespoonsful milk	6 tablespoonsful milk
2 teaspoonsful potato flour	2 teaspoonsful potato flour
Grated nutmeg	Grated nutmeg
½ teaspoonful yeast extract	½ teaspoonful yeast extract
2 tablespoonsful double cream	2 tablespoonsful heavy cream

1. Clean the mushrooms and slice thinly.
2. Cook gently in milk for about 10 minutes until tender.
3. Mix the potato flour with a little cold milk and add to mushrooms to thicken.
4. Season to taste, add a grating of nutmeg (this has a magical effect on the flavour of the mushrooms), the yeast extract and the cream.
5. Fill the potato hollows, reheat and brown under the grill (broiler). Serve with a green salad or just mustard and cress.

BAKED POTATOES WITH CREAM CHEESE AND HERBS

Serves 4

Imperial (Metric)	*American*
4 medium potatoes	4 medium potatoes
8 oz (225g) cream cheese	1 cupful cream cheese
2 tablespoonsful yogurt	2 tablespoonsful yogurt
Pinch sea salt	Pinch sea salt
Pinch paprika	Pinch paprika
Chopped chives, tarragon or savory or any other fresh chopped herbs	Chopped chives, tarragon or savory or any other fresh chopped herbs

1. Preheat the oven to 350°F/180°C (Gas Mark 4).
2. Scrub the potatoes thoroughly but do not peel.
3. Score once lengthways across the upper side of each potato and bake for 30-40 minutes.
4. While the potatoes are baking mix the cream cheese with the yogurt and add salt, paprika and chopped herbs to taste.
5. Remove the potatoes from the oven and arrange on a serving dish. Put the cream cheese mixture into a forcing bag and pipe over the slit in the baked potatoes.

BAKED POTATOES WITH CRISPY SKINS

Allow one medium-sized potato per person. Using a sharp knife, score slits across the back of the potato about ⅛-inch (3mm) apart. Season the slits and rub butter over them. Bake in the oven for about 40 minutes at 350°F/180°C (Gas Mark 4).

An unusual and delicious way of baking potatoes.

POTATO CAKES

Serves 4

Imperial (Metric)	*American*
1½ lbs (700g) potatoes	1½ pounds potatoes
4 tablespoonsful single cream	4 tablespoonsful light cream
1 egg yolk	1 egg yolk
Pinch sea salt	Pinch sea salt
¼ teaspoonful grated nutmeg	¼ teaspoonful grated nutmeg
1 tablespoonful chopped marjoram	1 tablespoonful chopped marjoram
1 tablespoonful chopped chives	1 tablespoonful chopped chives

1. Scrub the potatoes and steam or boil in their skins until cooked.
2. Drain the potatoes and remove their skins.
3. Mash thoroughly with cream and egg yolk adding salt to taste, nutmeg and herbs.
4. Form the mixture into rissoles or cakes and bake them on a greased baking tray in a hot oven 425°F/220°C (Gas Mark 7), until slightly browned. Serve with a mixed vegetable salad.

Variation:
Use 2 tablespoonsful sunflower seeds and 2 tablespoonsful chopped parsley instead of the chives or marjoram.

Vegetables

Most of the main dishes based on grains or potatoes in this section are fairly substantial and need only a green salad, dressed with a little olive oil, or some home grown mustard and cress, to accompany them.

If, however, a side dish of cooked vegetables is required it is best to serve one or two green vegetables that have been conservatively cooked either in just a little water (keep the liquor for vegetable stock) or, better still, steamed. A good steamer with dividers, so that more than one vegetable can be cooked at the same time, produces delicious vegetables that retain all their natural flavour and is very economical to use. Pressure cookers are not recommended for green vegetables; they tend to overcook however carefully they have been timed. All vegetables lend themselves to steaming and the larger ones can be sliced or chopped before cooking to shorten the cooking time.

The following vegetables are particularly good steamed:

- Asparagus tips (keep the stems to make asparagus soup — page 216).
- Tiny Brussels sprouts served with a little butter and topped with flaked almonds.
- Young runner (green) or french (snap) beans.
- Broccoli or calabrese spears.
- Spring carrots.
- Sliced aubergine (eggplant).
- Celery (cut into short lengths to steam and served with a little butter).
- Cauliflower florets.
- Small onions steamed whole or larger ones sliced.
- Fresh garden peas steamed with a sprig of mint and served with butter.

- Sliced parsnips, steamed and served with a little butter.
- Vegetable spaghetti (noodle squash) or any other type of marrow (squash).

Any left-over vegetables prepared in this way retain plenty of flavour and can be incorporated into a vegetable soup the next day.

16.

DESSERTS

BANANA CREAM

Serves 4

Imperial (Metric)	American
2 large *or* 3 small bananas	2 large *or* 3 small bananas
¼ pint (150ml) natural yogurt	⅔ cupful natural yogurt
¼ pint (150ml) whipping cream	⅔ cupful whipping cream
Sunflower seeds	Sunflower seeds

1. Blend the bananas in a liquidizer and mix well with the yogurt.
2. Whip the cream until stiff and fold into the banana mixture.
3. Serve in individual glasses topped with a scattering of sunflower seeds.

DATE ICE CREAM

Serves 4

Imperial (Metric)	*American*
16 pitted dates	16 pitted dates
8 fl oz (225ml) water	1 cupful water
1 tablespoonful spray-dried skimmed milk powder	1 tablespoonful spray-dried skimmed milk powder
¼ pint (150ml) whipping cream	⅔ cupful whipping cream

1. Put the dates in a blender. Add the water and dried milk powder and blend until smooth.
2. Whip the cream until stiff and fold into the date mixture.
3. Place in a container, cover with foil and freeze until firm.
4. Remove from the freezer and beat with a fork to ensure a smooth texture, and re-freeze.

GINGER BANANAS

Serves 4

Imperial (Metric)	*American*
4 ripe bananas	4 ripe bananas
A little preserved ginger	A little preserved ginger
Flaked almonds	Slivered almonds

1. Slice the bananas into individual dishes (one per person).
2. Rinse the syrup from the preserved ginger and chop fairly finely.
3. Sprinkle ginger over the bananas and top with a few almonds. Serve with a little whipped cream.

Variation:
Another way to serve bananas is to slice them as above, mix in a few drops of lemon juice (permissible because so little is used) to stop them going brown, and sprinkle with sunflower seeds.

EGG CUSTARD

Serves 2

Imperial (Metric)	*American*
6 fl oz (175ml) milk	¾ cupful milk
2 egg yolks	2 egg yolks
Mild honey to taste	Mild honey to taste
A few drops of *real* vanilla essence (optional)	A few drops of *real* vanilla essence (optional)

1. Heat the milk to boiling point and add slowly to the well-beaten egg yolks.
2. Return to the pan, preferably a double boiler, and stir over a gentle heat until the mixture thickens slightly.
3. Sweeten to taste with a mild-flavoured honey and add a few drops of vanilla essence if liked. The custard will thicken as it cools.

Variation:

FIG CUSTARD

1. Make an egg custard as above.
2. With kichen scissors snip dried figs into thin slices. Place in individual glasses and sprinkle over some finely chopped preserved ginger (any sugar adhering can be washed off), allowing a scant teaspoonful per serving. Top with the custard and decorate with whipped cream and/or chopped nuts of choice.

More Dessert Ideas for Starch Meals

● Sliced *fresh* figs in season — good alone or with a little thin cream.
● Fresh dates stuffed with freshly shelled walnuts.
● Date chips (obtainable from Wholefood Ltd., 24 Paddington Street, London, W.1.).
● Very sweet ripe pears sliced and served with a little thin cream.
● Frozen bananas: simply peel one banana per person to be served and put into the freezer as it is. When frozen solid, remove and put into the refrigerator for half an hour. Serve with a sprinkling of nuts and you have banana ice cream!
● Baked pears with raisins. Peel and halve very ripe dessert pears. Place in a baking dish with a scattering of raisins and a little water. Bake in the oven — 350°F/180°C (Gas Mark 4) — for about 20 minutes.

BREAD

This book would not be complete without giving the recipe for the delicious and easy no-kneading Grant loaf.

Since it was first published in *Your Daily Bread* (Faber, 1944) it has introduced countless families to the pleasure of eating really good wholewheat bread. It has also acquired a few variations which are included here.

You will not, however, find any recipes for cakes or biscuits as they have no place in the Hay system except for *very* occasional use. For the odd indulgence the authors heartily recommend *The Cranks Recipe Book* by David Canter, Kay Canter and Daphne Swann (J.M. Dent & Sons Ltd., 1982) which contains excellent sections on Cakes and Scones, Biscuits and Bread and many mouth-watering recipes for soups, salads and main dishes that can be adapted for the Hay system.

For people who are allergic to gluten, *The Sunday Times Book of Real Bread* (Rodale Press, 1982) gives many good bread recipes that offer a healthy alternative to the wholewheat loaf and Hilda Cherry Hill's book *Good Food Gluten Free* (Roberts Publications, 1976) offers many helpful recipes and ideas for coping with this problem. A more recent book, *The Complete Wheat-Free Cookbook* by Dr Sheila Gibson, Louise Templeton and Dr Robin Gibson (Thorsons, 1990), offers practical suggestions for following wheat-free diets with many delicious recipes for using oats, barley, rye and other grains. The recipes in this book are not all gluten-free but they *are* wheat-free. Dr Sheila Gibson considers that many clinical symptoms can be caused by wheat-sensitivity which seems to be not an allergy but a toxicity. The wheat toxicity-syndrome includes heart problems, high blood pressure, anxiety, migraine and many gastro-intestinal problems. Since wheat is sprayed with pesticides and herbicides many times during the course of its production this can be the reason why many people show symptoms of sensitivity to wheat, but not to other grains even though these may contain gluten. In a recent article in *Homoeopathy Today* Dr Gibson endorses the Hay principle of separating protein foods from carbohydrate foods because of its benefits for people with digestive problems.

Note: All the following bread recipes freeze well.

THE GRANT LOAF

Imperial (Metric)	*American*
3 lbs (1.35kg) stone ground wholewheat flour	12 cupsful stone ground wholewheat flour
2 teaspoonsful or less sea salt	2 teasponsful or less sea salt
2 pints (1.2 litres) water at blood heat (98.4°F/37°C)	5 cupsful water at blood heat (98.4°F/37°C)
3 level teaspoonsful dried yeast	3 level teaspoonsful dried yeast
2 level teaspoonsful Barbados sugar, honey or black molasses	2 level teaspoonsful Barbados sugar, honey or black molasses

1. Mix the salt with the flour (in very cold weather warm flour slightly to take off the chill).
2. Place 3 tablespoonsful of the water in a cup, sprinkle the dried yeast on top and leave for 2 minutes.
3. Add the sugar, honey or molasses. Leave for a further 10-15 minutes by which time there should be a thick creamy froth.
4. Make a well in the centre of the flour and pour in the yeast mixture and the rest of the water.
5. Mix well — by hand is best — for a minute or so, working from sides to middle until the dough feels elastic and leaves the side of the mixing bowl clean. Flours tend to vary in how much water they take up — the dough should be slippery.
6. Divide the dough into three 2 pint (1 litre/5 cup) bread tins which have been warmed and greased.
7. Put the tins in a warm (not hot) place, cover with a clean cloth and leave for about 20 minutes *or until the dough is within ½ inch (1cm) of the top of the tins*.
8. Bake in a fairly hot oven, 400°F/200°C (Gas Mark 6), for 35 to 40 minutes. If the loaf sounds hollow when the top is knocked, it is done.

Quantities for one loaf:

Imperial (Metric)	*American*
1 lb (450g) stoneground wholewheat flour	4 cupsful stoneground wholewheat flour
½ teaspoonful sea salt	½ teaspoonful sea salt
13-14 fl oz (360ml) water at blood heat (98.4°F/37°C)	1¾ cupsful water at blood heat (98.4°F/37°C)
1½ level teaspoonful dried yeast	1½ level teaspoonsful dried yeast
1 teaspoonful Barbados sugar, honey or black molasses	1 teaspoonful Barbados sugar, honey or black molasses

Variations on the Grant Loaf:

THE BRAN-PLUS LOAF

1. Substitute 1½ oz (40g/⅓ cupful) fresh unprocessed bran for 1½ oz (40g/⅓ cupful) wholewheat flour in every pound (450/4 cupsful)
2. Method — as for the Grant loaf.

THE GORDON GRANT LOAF

1. Substitute 1 oz (25g/¼ cupful) medium cut oatmeal for 1 oz (25g/¼ cupful) wholewheat flour in every pound (450g/4 cupsful)
2. Before baking the loaves sprinkle with sesame seeds thickly on top of the dough and press them down gently to make them adhere.
3. Method — as for the Grant loaf.

Note: The oatmeal enhances the lovely nutty flavour of the bread and increases its moisture-keeping quality.
  (This is what my husband has done to my loaf! — D.G.)

OVEN WHOLEWHEAT FLATTIES

1. Keep back some of the dough when making your bread. Place heaped tablespoonsful on to a greased baking sheet, leaving ample room between them.
2. With floured hands, press the spoonfuls into flat rounds — as flat as you can make them. Allow to rise until nicely puffed, then bake for about 20 minutes at bread temperature until a pale golden brown on top and crisp underneath.
3. These can be eaten as soon as they are cold; consisting mainly of well cooked 'outside' they are not indigestible like new bread can be. To serve, slit them open horizontally, remove any doughy inside, butter both halves and fill with various mixtures, such as egg and cress, honey and chopped parsley, or lettuce with a mixture of chopped fresh herbs. They are delicious eaten soon after they are cool, but not good if kept till the next day.

OATCAKES

Imperial (Metric)	*American*
5 oz (150g) medium cut oatmeal	1 cupful medium cut oatmeal
4 fl oz (125ml) boiling water	½ cupful boiling water
½ level teaspoonful sea salt	½ level teaspoonful sea salt
1 level teaspoonful unsalted butter	1 level teaspoonful unsalted butter

1. Preheat the oven to 350°F/180°C (Gas Mark 4).
2. Put the oatmeal into a mixing bowl.
3. Using a *Pyrex* jug, pour the boiling water over the sea salt and unsalted butter to melt them, add to the oatmeal and mix well.
4. Leave for a minute or so until the oatmeal swells and becomes workable.
5. Turn the mixture onto a well-floured pastry board and form into two equal-sized balls.
6. Roll out each ball separately into a small round and then cut this across four times to make eight wedge-shaped pieces.
7. Roll out each wedge as thinly as possible rolling from cut edge to cut edge —not from the outer edge to the point — in order to make nicely shaped pieces.
8. Place on a baking sheet and bake until cooked, when the wedges will be slightly curved, and a light golden colour on the edges. When cool, store in an airtight container.

Note: These oatcakes are delicious and quite different from factory made ones. Make sure that the oatmeal smells, and tastes, really *fresh*. Stale oatmeal tastes slightly bitter.

OATMEAL PORRIDGE

Just as quick as the instant kind but far more delicious.

Serves 2

Imperial (Metric)	*American*
4 oz (100g) medium cut oatmeal	1 cupful medium cut oatmeal
1 pint (550ml) water	2½ cupsful water
Pinch of sea salt	Pinch of sea salt

1. Bring the water to a boil in a thick-bottomed saucepan.
2. Stir in the oatmeal and cook at just under boiling point for 3 minutes, when the porridge will start to thicken.
3. Add sea salt to taste and pour into porridge bowls. As it cools slightly the porridge will thicken to the right consistency.
4. Serve with milk or top-of-the-milk cream.

Note: It is a good idea to sprinkle the porridge with raw oatmeal just before serving. This ensures that the porridge is well chewed rather than just swallowed — chewing is very important for starch digestion.

SANDWICH FILLINGS FOR PACKED MEALS

Use a genuine wholewheat bread such as the Grant loaf, or wholewheat rolls which are quicker and easier to prepare than cutting sandwiches.

Suggestions for fillings

- Mashed dates with grated lemon or orange rind.
- Dates and chopped celery.
- Dates and roughly chopped walnuts.
- Sliced tomatoes and lettuce leaves with chopped chives.
- Sliced cucumber and cress.
- Mustard and cress with savoury butter (butter flavoured with a little yeast extract), or sesame seed spread.
- Cress with cottage or cream cheese — but not a hard cheese such as Cheddar; even the soft cheeses constitute a compromise.
- Mashed bananas with chopped cashew nuts or almonds.
- Cream cheese with chopped fresh herbs.
- Mashed banana with chopped fresh parsley.
- Cold scrambled egg yolks with cress.
- Mashed cooked peas with a little chopped mint.
- Any mixed salad greens available with savoury butter.
- Cold French (snap) beans mashed with chopped hard-boiled egg yolk.

Any of the above sandwiches preceded by a vacuum flask of hot vegetable soup and followed by a handful of nuts and raisins or sunflower seeds would make an excellent and sustaining meal.

APPENDIX

ACID AND ALKALI-FORMING FOODS

A balanced diet consists of 20 per cent acid-forming foods to 80 per cent of alkali-forming foods.

The Acid-forming Foods

Meat (all kinds) including meat broths, extracts and soups

Poultry and game

Fish (all kinds) and shellfish

Cheese

Eggs

All grains, wheat, rice, oats, barley, buckwheat and grain products, except millet

Bread (all kinds)

Breakfast cereals (all kinds)

Flours of all kinds especially white flour

Sugar of all kinds and all products containing it, e.g.; jams and preserves, biscuits, pastries, soft drinks, cola drinks and commercial ice cream.

Beans, e.g., broad (Windsor), haricot (navy), flageolet, kidney and soya beans

Peas (dried)

Legumes: lentils, chick peas (Garbanzos), peanuts and peanut butter (not recommended)

Walnuts, cashews and pecans

Note: Wholegrain products such as 100% wholewheat flour and brown rice are less acid forming than white flour or polished rice. Condiments, pickles, sauces and vinegar are all acid forming also tea, coffee and alcohol. Seeds such as sunflower, sesame and pumpkin may be regarded as neutral.

Neutral Foods

Dairy Products

Milk — preferably raw — *not boiled or sterilized**
Buttermilk
Yogurt
Kefir
Fresh cream
Cream cheese

*Milk is a food for young mammals and should always be
used sparingly by adults. It should be regarded as a food, not
a drink and should not be served at a meal containing meat.
It should be used only in moderation with cereals and
starches.

When heat treated milk becomes more or less acid-forming
according to the degree of heat supplied.

Fats

Butter and vegetable oils such as olive, sunflower seed,
safflower and sesame seed oils are regarded as neutral.

The Alkali-forming Foods

Fruits

Apples
Apricots (fresh or dried)
Bananas
Cherries
Currants — red, black or
   white, *if ripe*
Dates
Figs (fresh or dried)
Gooseberries *if ripe*
Grapefruit
Grapes
Kiwis

Lemons
Mangoes
Melons
Nectarines
Oranges
Papayas
Peaches
Pears
Pineapple (fresh)
Prunes — Santa Clara
   prunes only
Raisins — all kinds
Raspberries
Strawberries

Nuts

Almonds
Brazil nuts
Chestnuts
Hazelnuts
Pine kernels (Pignolias)

Grains

Millet

Vegetables

Asparagus
Aubergines (eggplants)
Avocados
Beetroot (beet)
Broccoli
Brussels sprouts
Cabbage — all types
Calabrese
Carrots
Cauliflower
Celeriac
Celery
Chives
Courgettes (zucchini)
Cucumber
Dandelion leaves
Endive/chicory
Fresh green peas
Kale
Kohlrabi
Leeks
Lettuce
Marrow (squash)
Mushrooms
Mustard and cress
Onions
Parsnips
Peppers, green and red
Potatoes in skins
Radishes
Runner or string beans
(fresh)
Salsify
Seakale
Spinach
Spring greens
Spring onions (scallions)
Swedes (rutabagas)
Tomatoes
Turnips
Watercress

*It is impossible to list all fruits, but as a general guide all can be taken as being alkali-forming.

FURTHER READING

Health and Nutrition

Nutrition and Health, Sir Robert McCarrison & H.M. Sinclair, (McCarrison Society, 1982)

The Saccharine Disease, T.L. Cleave, (John Wright & Sons Ltd., Bristol, 1974)

How to Live Longer and Feel Better, Linus Pauling, (W.H. Freeman & Co., 1986)

Don't Forget Fibre in Your Diet, Denis Burkitt, M.D., F.R.C.S., F.R.S. (Martin Dunitz, 1979)

Taking the Rough with the Smooth, Dr Andrew Stanway, (Pan 1981)

A New Health Era, William Howard Hay, (Harrap: out of print but secondhand copies may be obtainable from secondhand bookshops)

Your Daily Food — Recipe for Survival, Doris Grant, (Faber & Faber, 1973)

The Food and Health of Western Man, Dr James Lambert Mount, (Charles Knight, 1975)

Choose Health, Choose Life, Kenneth Vickery, (Kingsway Publications Ltd., 1986)

The Right Way to Eat, Miriam Polunin, (J.M. Dent, 1978)

The Pritikin Promise, Nathan Pritikin, (Bantam, 1985)

The Food Factor, Barbara Griggs, (Penguin, 1989)

Zest for Life, Barbara Griggs, (Ebury Press, 1989)

Effects of Western Food & Environment

The Role of Medicine: Dream, Mirage or Nemesis, Thomas McKeown, (Nuffield Prov. Hosp. Trust, 1976)

The Diseases of Civilisation, Brian Inglis, (Hodder & Stoughton, 1981)

Cured to Death — The Effects of Prescription Drugs, Arabella Melville & Colin Johnson, (Secker & Warburg, 1982)

Health Shock, Martin Weitz, (David & Charles, 1980)

Living Dangerously, Hilda Cherry Hills, (Roberts Publications, 1986)

Cover Up — The Facts They Don't Want You to Know, Nicholas Hildyard, (New English Library, 1981)

Diet, Crime and Delinquency, Alexander Schauss, (Parker House, Ca., 1980)

Food Irradiation: the Myth and the Reality, Tony Webb & Tim Lang, (Thorsons, 1990)

Food for Nought — The Decline in Nutrition, Ross Hume Hall, (Harper & Row, 1974)

Food Additives and Your Health, Beatrice Trum Hunter, (Keats, 1972)

Pure, White & Deadly, The Problem of Sugar, John Yudkin, (Penguin, 1988)

The Food Scandal, Caroline Walker & Geoffrey Cannon, (Century Arrow, 1986)

Allergy and Related Problems

Why Your Child is Hyperactive, Ben F. Feingold, M.D., (Random House, N.Y., 1975)

Not All in the Mind, Richard Mackarness, (Pan, 1990)

Chemical Victims, Richard Mackarness, (Pan 1980)

Eating and Allergy, Robert Eagle, (Thorsons, 1986)

The Allergy Connection, Barbara Paterson, (Thorsons, 1985)

Chemical Children, Dr Peter Mansfield & Dr Jean Monro, (Century, 1987)

The Migraine Revolution, Dr John Mansfield, (Thorsons, 1986)

Arthritis — The Allergy Connection, Dr John Mansfield, (Thorsons, 1990)

Eating for Health: Wholefood Cookbooks

The New Cookbook, Miriam Polunin, (Macdonald, 1984)
The Healthy Gourmet, Caroline Waldegrave, (Grafton, 1986)
Fresh Thoughts on Food, Lynda Brown, (Dorling Kindersley, 1988)
Good Housekeeping Wholefood Cookery, Gail Duff, (Ebury Press, 1980)
High Fibre Cooking, Janette Marshall, (Thorsons, 1983)
The High Fibre Cookbook, Pamela Westland, (Martin Dunitz, 1982)
Jane Grigson's Vegetable Book, (Penguin, 1980)
Sugar Off!, Richard & Elizabeth Cook, (Great Ouse Press, 1983)
The Sunday Times Book of Real Bread, Michael Bateman & Heather Maisner, (Rochdale Press Inc., 1982)

Vegetarian Cookbooks

The Bristol Recipe Book, Sadhya Rippon, (Century, 1987)
The Cranks Recipe Book, David & Kay Canter and Daphne Swann, (J.M. Dent, 1982)
Entertaining with Cranks, David & Kay Canter and Daphne Swann, (J.M. Dent, 1985)
Any books by Rose Elliot, but in particular:
   Gourmet Vegetarian Cooking, (Fontana, 1983)
   Supreme Vegetarian Cookery Book, (Fontana, 1990)
   The Green Age Diet, (Fontana, 1990)
The Bircher-Benner Health Guide, Ruth Kunz-Bircher, (George Allen & Unwin, 1981)
Eating Your Way to Health, Ruth Bircher & Claire Loewenfeld, (Faber & Faber, 1966)
Eastern Vegetarian Cookery, Madhur Jaffrey, (Cape, 1983)
Cordon Vert, Colin Spencer, (Thorsons, 1985)
Mediterranean Vegetarian Cooking, Colin Spencer, (Thorsons, 1986)
The Winter Vegetarian, Stephanie Segal, (Papermac, 1989)

Macrobiotics

The Book of Whole Meals, Annemarie Colbin, (Ballantine Books N.Y., 1983)
The Complete Wheat-free Cookbook, Sheila L.M. Gibson, Louise Templeton & Robin Gibson, (Thorsons, 1990)
The Practically Macrobiotic Cookbook, Keith Michell, (Thorsons, 1987)

Food Combining

Good Foods that Go Together, Esther L. Smith, (Keats, 1975)
Food Combining Cookbook, Erwina Lidolt, (Thorsons, 1987)
The Biogenic Diet, Leslie Kenton, (Century, 1986)
The Wright Diet, Celia Wright, (Piatkus, 1986)

Raw Foods, Herbs and Salads

Raw Energy, Leslie & Susannah Kenton, (Century, 1984)
Raw Energy Recipes, Leslie & Susannah Kenton, (Century, 1985)
The Raw Food Way to Health, Janet Hunt, (Thorsons, 1978)
Herbs for Health & Cookery, Claire Loewenfeld & Philippa Back, (Pan, 1965)
A Herb Cookbook, Gilian Painter, (Hodder & Stoughton, 1983)
The Home Herbal, Barbara Griggs, (Pan, 1986)
The Cook's Garden, Lynda Brown, (Century, 1990)

Growing Your Own

Culinary and Salad Herbs, Eleanor Sinclair Rohde, (Dover Publications Inc., 1972)
The Salad Garden, Joy Larkcom, (Windward, 1984)
Salads the Year Round, Joy Larkcom, (Hamlyn, 1980)

Directories: Where to Find Wholefood and Organic Suppliers

Shopping for Health, Janette Marshall, (Penguin, 1987)
International Vegetarian Handbook 1989/1990 (The Vegetarian Society, Parkdale, Dunham Road, Altrincham, Cheshire)
Thorsons Organic Consumer Guide, Edited by David Mabey and Alan & Jackie Gear, (Thorsons, 1990)

Note: All the cookbooks listed above contain excellent recipes that can be adapted to the Hay system and are particularly helpful in providing new ideas for the preparation of salads, fruit and vegetables.

In case of difficulty, most of them can be obtained from the Wholefood Bookshop, 24 Paddington Street, London W1M 4DR.

USEFUL ADDRESSES

For information about local wholefood and organic suppliers consult *Thorsons Organic Consumer Guide* edited by David Mabey and Alan and Jackie Gear (Thorons, 1990), or contact The National Centre for Organic Gardening, Ryton-on-Dunsmore, Coventry, CV8 3LG.

In case of difficulty the following wholefood and organic suppliers have a mail order service. Send s.a.e. for price lists.

Wholefoods
Biodynamic Products, Caradoc Ltd, Caradoc House, 121 Bath Road, Worcester WR5 3AF. (Suppliers of excellent biodynamically grown grains, cereals and herb teas and biodynamic skin care preparations.)
Real Foods, 37 Broughton Street, Edinburgh, EH1 3JU. (Also carries an excellent range of herbs and spices.)
Sunfood, 5 Bear Street, Barnstaple, Devon.
Freshlands Wholefoods, 196 Old Street, London EC1V 9BP (send first class s.a.e.)
Wholefood Ltd., 24 Paddington Street, London W1M 4DR.
Wholefoods, Unit 2D, Kylmore Industrial Estate, Killeen, Dublin 10.

Teas, Herb Teas, Herbs and Spices
Culpeper Ltd., Hadstock Road, Linton, Cambridge CB1 6NJ.
L'Herbier de Provence, 341 Fulham Road, London SW10.
Brazilian Yerbama Co. Ltd., Lamerton, Tavistock, Devon PL19 8RN. (Pure maté tea free of all added flavourings and chemicals.)

Organic Honey Suppliers
Pure Honey Supplies Co., Mildon House, Cedar Avenue, Enfield, Middlesex.
Organic Food Service, Ashe, Churston Ferrers, Brixham, S. Devon.

Allergy and Hyperactivity
Hyperactive Children's Support Group, 71 Whyke Lane, Chichester, W. Sussex, PO19 2LD.
(Much practical advice and help; details of the Feingold diet and 'safe' foods list; regular newsletter containing useful information which is constantly updated.)
   Secretary: Sally Bunday — send s.a.e. to above address for details.

Information on additives can be obtained from *E for Additives* by Maurice Hanssen (Thorsons, 1987) or The Ministry of Agriculture, Publications Unit, Lion House, Willowburn Trading Estate, Alnwick, Northumberland, NE66 2PF.

Food and Supplements for Exclusion and Special Diets
The Cantassium Co. Ltd., 225 Putney Bridge Road, London SW15 2PY.
For information about local wholefood and organic suppliers consult: *'The Organic Network'*, edited by Jean Winter, published by Eden Acres, Inc, 1984. Updated annually. Available from: Eden Acres, Inc, 12100 Lima Center Road, Clinton, Michigan 49236. Tel: (517) 456-4288.

Mailorder Services for Wholefoods and Organic Supplies:
Walnut Acres, Penns Creek, Pennsylvania 17862. Tel: (717) 837-0601.
The Good Food Store, 920 Kensington, Missoula, Montana 59801. Tel: (406) 728-5823.

Eden's Foods, 701 Tecumseh Road, Clinton, Michigan 49236. Tel: (517) 456-7424.
Kahan and Lessin Distributors, 3131 E. Maria Street, Compton, California 90221. Tel: (213) 631-5121.

Teas, Herb Teas, Herbs, and Spices
Aphrodesia Products, 45 Washington Street, Brooklyn, New York 11201.
Biobotanica Inc, 75 Commerce Drive, Hauppauge, New York 11788.
Green Mountain Herb Inc, 4890 Pear Street, Boulder, Colorado 80301.
San Francisco Herb, Tea and Spice Trading Company, 4543 Horton Street, Emery Ville, California 94601.
Sweethardt Herbs, Box 12602, Austin, Texas 78711.
The Whole Herb Company, 250 East Blithedale, Mill Valley, California 99494.
In Canada:
Lifestream, 12411 Volcan Way, Richmond, B.C., Canada V6V 1J7.
Wide World of Herbs, 11 Saint Catherine Street East, Montreal 129, Canada.

Organic Honey Suppliers
Draper's Super Bee Apiaries, R.D.1, Box 97, Millerton, Pennsylvania 16936. Tel: (800) 233-4273.
Francis and Elizabeth Bradac, Ramblewood Acres, 985 Englewood Avenue, St. Paul, Minnesota 55104.

Allergy, Hyperactivity, and Nutrition
Allergy Foundation of America, 801 2nd Avenue, New York, New York 10017. (Fosters research in allergic reactions to food.)
International College of Applied Nutrition, P.O. Box 386, La Habra, California 90631. (Specializes in nutritional aspects of disease.)
National Academy of Sciences, 2101 Constitution Avenue N.W., Washington, D.C. 20418. Tel: (202) 334-3318. (Up-

to-date information on additives, disease, and nutrition.)

Food and Drug Administration, Public Health Service, Department of Health, Education and Welfare, 5600 Fishers Lane, Rockville, Maryland 20857. Tel: (301) 443-3170.

Organic bran. Nicholas Terance, The Water Mill, Little Salkeld, Penrith, Cumbria. Tel: (076 881) 523.

INDEX

RECIPE INDEX

P = recipe for protein meal
S = recipe for starch meal